Acute Gynaecology and Early Pregnancy

Advanced Skills Series

Acute Gynaecology and Early Pregnancy

Advanced Skills Series

Edited by Davor Jurkovic and Roy Farquharson

WITHDRAWN

RCOG PRESS

A machine-readable catalogue record for this publication is available from the British Library [www.bl.uk/catalogue/listings.html]

ISBN 978-1-906985-32-5

Published by the RCOG Press at the Royal College of Obstetricians and Gynaecologists
27 Sussex Place, Regent's Park, London NW1 4RG

Registered Charity No. 213280

RCOG Press Editor: Claire Dunn
Indexer: Liza Furnival
Text & typesetting: Christopher Wakeling / Typographic Design Unit
Printed in the UK by Latimer Trend & Co. Ltd, Estover Road, Plymouth PL6 7PL

Contents

WITHDRAWN

About the authors

Willem M Ankum MD
Consultant, Department of Obstetrics and Gynaecology, Academic Medical Centre, University of Amsterdam, The Netherlands

Cecilia Bottomley MRCOG
Consultant Obstetrician and Gynaecologist, Chelsea and Westminster NHS Foundation Trust, London, UK

Christy Burden MRCOG
Specialist Registrar, Department of Obstetrics and Gynaecology, Southmead Hospital, Bristol, UK

T Justin Clark MRCOG
Consultant Obstetrician and Gynaecologist, Birmingham Women's Hospital, Birmingham, UK

Natalie AM Cooper MB ChB
Clinical Research Fellow, University of Birmingham, Birmingham Women's Hospital, Birmingham, UK

Caroline Cormack FRCA
Consultant Anaesthetist, Department of Anaesthesia, University College Hospital, London, UK

Natasha Curran FRCA
Consultant Anaesthetist, Department of Anaesthesia, University College Hospital, London, UK

Janine Elson FRCOG
Medical Director, Leicester Fertility Centre, and Consultant, University of Leicester, Leicester Royal Infirmary, Leicester, UK

Roy Farquharson FRCOG
Consultant in Obstetrics and Gynaecology, Liverpool Women's Hospital, Liverpool, UK

Petra J Hajenius MD PhD
Consultant Obstetrician and Gynaecologist, Department of Obstetrics and Gynaecology, Academic Medical Centre, University of Amsterdam, Amsterdam, The Netherlands

Jennifer Hopwood FFSRH, Dip Ven
Consultant in Contraception and Sexual Health, and Director of the Wirral Chlamydia Programme, St Catherine's Hospital, Birkenhead, UK (now retired)

Amna Jamil MBBS
Clinical Research Fellow, Department of Obstetrics and Gynaecology, University College Hospital, London, UK

Eric Jauniaux PhD FRCOG
Professor of Obstetrics and Fetal Medicine, Academic Department of Obstetrics and Gynaecology, University College London, London, UK

Davor Jurkovic FRCOG
Consultant Gynaecologist, Department of Obstetrics and Gynaecology, University College Hospital, London, UK

Emma Kirk MRCOG
Specialist Registrar in Obstetrics and Gynaecology, Whittington Hospital NHS Trust, London, UK

Femke Mol MD
Consultant Gynaecologist and Subspeciality Trainee in Reproductive Medicine, Centre for Reproductive Medicine, Department of Obstetrics and Gynaecology, Academic Medical Centre, University of Amsterdam, Amsterdam, The Netherlands

Caroline Overton FRCOG
Consultant Obstetrician and Gynaecologist, St Michael's University Hospital, Bristol, UK

Neelam Potdar MRCOG
Subspecialist Registrar in Reproductive Medicine, Leicester Fertility Centre,
and Clinical Lecturer, University of Leicester, Leicester Royal Infirmary,
Leicester, UK

Jackie Ross MRCOG
Consultant Gynaecologist, Early Pregnancy and Gynaecology Assessment
Unit, King's College Hospital, London, UK

Rehan Salim MRCOG
Consultant, Department of Obstetrics and Gynaecology, University College
Hospitals, London, UK

Sangeeta Suri MRCOG
Specialist Registrar, Department of Obstetrics and Gynaecology, University
College Hospital, London, UK

Michelle Swer BSc BA MBBCh BAO
Clinical Research Fellow, Department of Obstetrics and Gynaecology,
University College Hospital, London, UK

Norah M van Mello MD
Specialist Registrar in Obstetrics and Gynaecology, Academic Medical
Centre, University of Amsterdam, Amsterdam, The Netherlands

Sanjay Vyas FRCOG
Consultant Gynaecologist and Laparoscopic Surgeon, Department
of Obstetrics and Gynaecology, Southmead Hospital, Bristol, UK

Acknowledgements

Chapter 14

Natalie A M Cooper and T Justin Clark would like to thank Miss Maureen Dalton MRCS LRCP FRCOG, Consultant Obstetrician and Gynaecologist at Royal Devon and Exeter Hospital (Heavitree). The section on sexual assault was written after consultation with Miss Dalton.

Abbreviations

5-ASA	5 aminosalicyclic acid
5-HT3	5 hydroxytryptamine 3
ABC	airway, breathing and circulation
AEPU	Association of Early Pregnancy Units
ATSM	Advanced Training Skills Module
AVM	arteriovenous malformation
CA125	cancer antigen 125
CEMACH	Confidential Enquiry into Maternal and Child Health
CHM	complete hydatidiform mole
CI	confidence interval
CRL	crown–rump length
CRP	C-reactive protein
CT	computed tomography
CVP	central venous pressure
DDAVP	1-desamino-8-d-arginine vasopressin (desmopressin)
ERPC	evacuation of retained products of conception
hCG	human chorionic gonadotrophin
HG	hyperemesis gravidarum
HRT	hormone replacement therapy
IGFBP-1	insulin-like growth factor-binding protein 1
IVF	in vitro fertilisation
LFT	liver function test
LSD	d-lysergic acid diethylamide
MRI	magnetic resonance imaging
MSU	mid-stream urine
NAAT	nucleic acid amplification test
NEAD study	Neurodevelopmental Effects of Antiepileptic Drugs study
NICE	National Institute for Health and Clinical Excellence
NSAID	non-steroidal anti-inflammatory drug
PEACH study	PID Evaluation And Clinical Health study
PHM	partial hydatidiform mole
PID	pelvic inflammatory disease
PTD	persistent trophoblastic disease

RR	relative risk
TEDS	thromboembolic-deterrent stockings
TFT	thyroid function test
TMP-SMX	trimethoprim–sulphonamide
TPN	total parenteral nutrition
TSH	thyroid-stimulating hormone
TVS	transvaginal sonography
UCHL	University College Hospital, London

Preface

Acute gynaecological problems are among the most common reasons for women of reproductive age to seek medical help. Early pregnancy complications account for the majority of gynaecological emergencies. In the UK, emergency gynaecological care used to be provided mainly by junior doctors working in casualty departments. However, it became clear that this model of care was not well suited to meeting the needs and increasing expectations of women. Developments in diagnostic ultrasound, which occurred in parallel, have led to wide acceptance of ultrasound as an essential tool for the assessment of developing pregnancy from a very early stage until delivery. Routine ultrasound scanning to assess fetal health and wellbeing has now been introduced in most developed countries.

To meet demands for more accessible, patient-centred care, early pregnancy assessment units were developed in the UK. This model of care has proved to be very successful and has been adopted by most acute hospitals. Early pregnancy units usually provide an integrated ultrasound scanning service to facilitate diagnostic work-up and to formulate appropriate management plans. Easier access to health professionals with an interest in early pregnancy care and greater availability of ultrasound scanning have resulted in increased attendance at early pregnancy units, with many women wishing to confirm that their pregnancy is normal rather than seeking help for serious medical complications. Improved diagnosis of miscarriage and ectopic pregnancy has prompted the development and implementation of more conservative management strategies. As a result, the number of follow-up visits has increased, contributing further to high attendance rates. In many hospitals, emergency outpatient visits now outnumber elective clinic appointments in gynaecology.

In the UK, the majority of early pregnancy care is delivered by nurses and sonographers, who are typically supported only by junior trainees in obstetrics and gynaecology with little or no input from senior medical staff. With the rising number of patients, the increased complexity of diagnostic algorithms and a wide range of available management options, it has become increasingly clear that consultant participation in early pregnancy and acute gynaecological care is required to maintain and develop clinical standards. Although ultrasound examinations and blood tests often provide sufficient information to confidently diagnose and manage many acute gynaecological problems, in a significant proportion of women the results of such tests are not conclusive and the diagnosis remains unclear. In these cases, clinical assessment by experienced senior doctors is often the only way to ensure that management is rational and safe without subjecting women to unnecessary hospital admissions and operative investigations.

Until the late 2000s, doctors completing specialist training in the UK were ill prepared to provide a high-quality clinical service to women with acute gynaecological problems and early pregnancy complications. To address this gap in the training programme, the RCOG established an Advanced Training Skills Module for doctors who wish to develop further their skills in the management of gynaecological emergencies. This book provides a supporting reference text to trainees undertaking this advanced training in acute gynaecology; other medical professionals with an interest in emergency gynaecological care will also find it helpful. The authors are all recognised experts in the field of acute gynaecology and early pregnancy, and many of them run large acute gynaecology units in their hospitals. The authors' extensive clinical experience is reflected in the text, which contains a plethora of helpful practical advice and many illustrations, flow charts and diagrams which readers will find useful when trying to solve unfamiliar or complex problems in their daily practice.

In addition to chapters covering the diagnosis and management of routine clinical problems such as miscarriage and tubal pregnancy, there are chapters on uncommon forms of ectopic pregnancy and trophoblastic disease. Although these problems are relatively rare, they are associated with increased maternal morbidity and it is essential that those involved in providing early pregnancy care are familiar with their diagnosis and management. We have also included a large chapter on drugs in early pregnancy. Pregnant women are often concerned about possible adverse effects of drugs on their unborn babies. This chapter will be helpful when counselling women regarding risks associated with various medications.

We are all aware that theoretical knowledge gathered from books and other sources of written information can provide only the fundamentals for developing good clinical practice. Caring for women with early pregnancy and acute gynaecological problems also requires sound clinical judgement and excellent communication skills, which can be developed only by practising in busy acute units. Greater emphasis on acute gynaecological care within the trainees' curriculum could represent the first step towards establishing a new subspecialty in acute gynaecology and early pregnancy care. This book, by providing a comprehensive review of many novel and exciting developments in this field, will help to facilitate this process and attract more young doctors to this important and rewarding area of clinical practice.

Davor Jurkovic and Roy Farquharson

1

Organisation and delivery of emergency care in early pregnancy and acute gynaecology

Roy Farquharson and Caroline Overton

Introduction

Early pregnancy problems account for a major part of all gynaecological emergencies. Other less common gynaecological emergencies are acute pain, severe vaginal bleeding and collapse, which are covered in detail in other chapters.

All women with early pregnancy and acute gynaecological problems should receive prompt referral to a dedicated early pregnancy unit that provides efficient, evidence-based care with access to appropriate information and counselling. The National Service Framework recommends that all women should have access to an early pregnancy unit, which should be easily available (www.earlypregnancy.org.uk). Ideally, these services should also be directly accessible to GPs.

A report of the National Confidential Enquiry into Patient Outcome and Death in 2007 stated that when a patient with an acute healthcare problem arrives in hospital, he or she requires prompt clinical assessment, appropriate investigations and institution of a clear management plan. There should be an early decision regarding the need to involve all relevant specialties and other required services followed by a timely review by an appropriately trained senior clinician. This should be undertaken in an environment that is best suited to meet the patient's clinical needs. Although there is conflicting opinion on the optimal location for the assessment of emergency admissions, it has been recommended that women presenting with early pregnancy complications should undergo initial assessment in dedicated emergency assessment units. The rationale for the use of emergency assessment units is that they can reduce both the emergency department's workload and hospital length of stay. Patients can be seen sooner by a senior doctor, which will result in earlier decision making and so expedite treatment. This may improve patient outcome and satisfaction. Standards set by the Society for Acute Medicine state that there should be a designated lead clinician and clinical manager in charge of an emergency assessment unit.

At all times, women should be supported in making informed choices about their care and management. Easy-to-read information leaflets should supplement these choices. Appropriate follow-up systems should be in place to facilitate repeat scans or blood tests.

Early pregnancy units should be encouraged to work collaboratively to share good practice and participate in clinical audit and research to improve standards of care for all women with problems in early pregnancy. Feedback from support organisations such as the Miscarriage Association, the Ectopic Pregnancy Trust and the Association of Early Pregnancy Units (AEPU) suggests that women want prompt and sensitive treatment of early pregnancy problems as well as a full explanation of management choices, which should be supplemented with easy-to-read information leaflets.

In the past, pregnant women were admitted to the emergency receiving ward and waited for a considerable length of time before undergoing ultrasound scan and clinical assessment. With the appearance of early pregnancy units, an increasing number of women are being assessed and managed as outpatients or office attenders. The advent of high-resolution transvaginal ultrasound coupled with improved access to serum human chorionic gonadotrophin (hCG) measurements has allowed the development of models of care and improved the delivery of care.

In the UK, the number of early pregnancy units has increased rapidly and over 200 active units are now registered with the AEPU. The AEPU has set out, since its inception in 2001, to improve the standards of early pregnancy care and to provide a clearer pathway for the patient's journey (www.early pregnancy.org.uk).

The mission statement from the AEPU puts the woman at the centre of all activity, and the multidisciplinary care structure reflects the multi-tasking approach of care providers: 'All women with early pregnancy problems will have prompt access to a dedicated early pregnancy assessment unit that provides efficient management, counselling and access to appropriate information. At all times women will be supported in making informed choices about their care and management.'

In the UK, there are approximately 700 000 births, 200 000 terminations of pregnancy, more than 250 000 miscarriages and 15 000 ectopic pregnancies per annum.[1] In addition to this huge activity profile there are clear trends, including increasing maternal age, increasing demand for and access to acute gynaecological services, increasing knowledge about early pregnancy events (approximately 17 500 000 entries on Google) and improved choice of care provider for pregnant women.

Standards of practice

Standards in early pregnancy care

In recent years, ultrasound diagnosis and improved understanding of problems related to early pregnancy have led to the introduction of medical and expectant management of miscarriage and selected cases of ectopic pregnancy. Randomised controlled trials have provided evidence-based practice (www.rcog.org.uk/guidelines). Patient choice has emerged as a powerful selector for treatment.

The opportunity is now here for clear core standards to be applied to harmonise care provision across the UK. The AEPU has constructed ten key points to lay down a solid foundation for care providers.[2] In conjunction with the RCOG and patient groups, including the Miscarriage Association and Ectopic Pregnancy Trust, as well as related professionals (especially psychologists), a set of standards has been published on early pregnancy care, ectopic pregnancy and recurrent miscarriage (Table 1.1).[3,4]

Standards in ectopic pregnancy

Ectopic pregnancy can sometimes cause serious complications and women should receive prompt referral to a dedicated early pregnancy unit providing efficient management and patient counselling. Early pregnancy units should have a protocol in place for conducting a pregnancy test and transvaginal ultrasound in women of reproductive age with amenorrhoea associated with abdominal pain.[5] Access to serial serum hCG laboratory measurements is mandatory for efficient diagnosis, surveillance and monitoring. All units should have clear guidelines in place for the management of pregnancies of unknown location.[2] Table 1.2 outlines current standards in ectopic pregnancy.

Standards in recurrent miscarriage

Recurrent miscarriage is defined as three or more consecutive pregnancy losses and affects about 1% of couples. Maternal age and the number of previous losses are two important factors in determining future prognosis. Although the pathophysiology remains unknown in almost 50% of cases, structural uterine abnormalities, chromosomal anomalies and maternal thrombophilia have been directly associated with recurrent miscarriage.[3,6]

All early pregnancy units or recurrent miscarriage clinics should have a clearly defined protocol for the investigation of women with recurrent miscarriage. Table 1.3 outlines current standards in recurrent miscarriage.

TABLE 1.1 **Standards in early pregnancy care**

1 Patient focus	Women should be offered a range of management options with a full explanation of the processes involved.
	There should be an appropriately furnished room for breaking bad news.
	All emotional and psychological counselling requirements should be provided within the EPU.
	There should be access to bereavement counselling.
	Clear patient information should be available on pathology tests, postmortem examination and sensitive disposal options.
2 Accessibility	All EPUs should offer a minimum service that includes a 5-day clinic opening during office hours with full staffing and scan support. Ideally, there should be a 7-day service.
	There should be direct referral for women with a history of recurrent pregnancy loss or previous ectopic pregnancy.
3 Environment	All EPUs should have a designated reception area constantly staffed during opening hours.
	There should be direct referral access for other healthcare professionals such as accident and emergency departments and NHS Direct/NHS24.
4 Process	All EPUs should offer a full range of options for managing both miscarriage and ectopic pregnancy (conservative, medical and surgical). Care pathways should be in place for each management option.
	Guidelines and algorithms should be in place for the management of: ○ pregnancy of uncertain viability ○ pregnancy of unknown location ○ suspected ectopic pregnancy.
	All EPUs should have laboratory access to serum hCG measurement, with blood group results available the same day. Ideally, blood group results should be available within 2 hours.
	All women undergoing surgical intervention for miscarriage should be offered screening test for *Chlamydia trachomatis*.
	Access to a daily serum progesterone assay as part of a clinical algorithm will facilitate management of cases of pregnancy of unknown location.
5 Audit	All EPUs should have regular clinical governance meetings to review clinical protocols and critical incidents and to assess the need for continuing training.
6 Staffing and competence	All EPUs should hold a register of staff competent in transabdominal and transvaginal scanning.
	All staff should undergo formal training in emotional and psychological support.
7 Auditable standards	All EPUs should audit patient choice and uptake rates for medical/surgical/conservative management of miscarriage, together with complications and failure rates.
	All EPUs should audit on an annual basis adherence to the RCOG Green-top Guideline No. 25: *The management of early pregnancy loss*.

EPU = early pregnancy unit | hCG = human chorionic gonadotrophin.

TABLE 1.2 **Standards in ectopic pregnancy**

1 Patient focus	All EPUs should provide patient information on all aspects of ectopic pregnancy diagnosis, management and future care, together with information on future fertility.
	All staff should be trained to provide emotional support to women who experience an ectopic pregnancy.
2 Accessibility	All EPUs should have a policy in place for referring women with suspected ectopic pregnancy from the primary care or accident and emergency setting directly to an EPU for immediate assessment or to the nearest gynaecology emergency ward.
	All EPUs should have a protocol in place to carry out a pregnancy test and transvaginal ultrasound in women of reproductive age presenting with any type of abdominal pain, irregular vaginal bleeding or amenorrhoea.
3 Process	All EPUs should accept self-referral from women with pain or bleeding in early pregnancy, especially those with a previous history of ectopic pregnancy.
	All primary care organisations should use one type of urinary pregnancy test to confirm or exclude pregnancy to reduce risk of error.
	All EPUs should have laboratory access to serum hCG measurement, with blood group results available the same day. Ideally, blood group results should be available within 2 hours.
	All EPUs should have in place clear guidelines for the management of pregnancies of unknown location, based on the RCOG Green-top Guideline No. 25: *The management of early pregnancy*. A clear explanation of surgical, medical and expectant management options should be given, depending on the clinical scenario and local availability.
	All EPUs should offer laparoscopic management of ectopic pregnancy in women who are haemodynamically stable, at least during normal working hours.
	All EPUs should offer medical treatment to suitable women, following a local protocol with methotrexate, but only in units where women can access 24-hour telephone advice and emergency admission if required.
	Women undergoing medical or expectant management for an ectopic pregnancy should have handheld notes documenting ultrasound findings, serum hCG levels, treatment given and follow-up serum hCG levels in case of need for emergency attendance out of hours or at another unit.
4 Audit and outcome	All units should audit patient choice and uptake rates for medical/surgical/conservative management of ectopic pregnancy, together with complications and failure rates.
	All units should audit on an annual basis adherence to the RCOG Green-top Guideline No. 21: *The management of tubal pregnancy*.
5 Staffing and competence	All gynaecologists should be proficient in the laparoscopic management of ectopic pregnancy. In the future, they should have completed an appropriate Advanced Training Skills Module.
6 Auditable standards	All units should audit patient choice and uptake rates of medical/surgical/conservative management of pregnancy of unknown location combined with outcome and complication rates, including surgical intervention.
	All units should audit on an annual basis adherence to the RCOG Green-top Guideline No. 21: *The management of tubal pregnancy*.
	All EPUs should record their incidence of ruptured ectopic pregnancy and of failed diagnosis of an unruptured ectopic pregnancy.

EPU = early pregnancy unit | hCG human chorionic gonadotrophin.

TABLE 1.3 **Standards in recurrent miscarriage**

1 Patient focus	Information leaflets should be available for women and their families on local referral pathways, investigation, management and future care.
	All women with a history of recurrent miscarriage should be offered a follow-up visit to discuss issues such as fertility and early management of subsequent pregnancies.
2 Accessibility	All women who present with known criteria for recurrent miscarriage should be offered advice and referred to an EPU/specialist clinic either locally or at a tertiary unit.
3 Environment	All women with recurrent miscarriage should have access to an EPU/miscarriage clinic with appropriately trained healthcare professionals.
	Arrangements should be in place for women with a future confirmed pregnancy test to attend an EPU for an ultrasound scan and to receive shared antenatal care in a high-risk obstetric clinic.
4 Process	There should be a clearly defined protocol for investigating couples with recurrent miscarriage as regards prenatal karyotyping, thrombophilia screening and infection screening.
	Couples should be informed that women whose ovaries have a polycystic appearance at ultrasound scan and who ovulate are not at increased risk of recurrent miscarriage and will not require anti-estrogen treatment.
	Three-dimensional ultrasound should be used for assessment of uterine malformations, as it may prevent the need for diagnostic hysteroscopy and laparoscopy.
	Cervical weakness should be considered only in women presenting with recurrent mid-trimester miscarriages.
	Preimplantation genetic screening has no place in the management of recurrent miscarriage.
	Each unit should have a care pathway in place for managing a diagnosis of recurrent mid-trimester loss as regards cervical cerclage and transvaginal assessment of cervical length.
	Thromboprophylaxis should be commenced with aspirin, with or without heparin, for women with antiphospholipid syndrome and thrombophilia from diagnosis of intrauterine pregnancy. Heparin should be continued for 6 weeks postpartum, with bone mineral density surveillance.
	Cytogenetic analysis of the products of conception should be considered only for women who have undergone treatment in the index pregnancy or are participants in a research trial.
5 Audit and outcome	All clinical staff should attend regular clinical governance meetings and a record should be maintained. Standard agenda items should include audit, adverse incidents, protocols and service development.
6 Staffing and competence	All recurrent miscarriage clinics should have in place a named consultant with a special interest in recurrent miscarriage.
	All recurrent miscarriage clinics should have multidisciplinary support from genetics, EPU, pathology, radiology and haematology departments.
	All staff dealing with recurrent miscarriage should be trained in emotional aspects of pregnancy loss to provide immediate support and to enable access to specialist counselling.
7 Auditable standards	All services should audit on an annual basis adherence to the RCOG Green-top Guideline No. 17: *The investigation and treatment of couples with recurrent miscarriage.*

EPU = early pregnancy unit.

Recurrent miscarriage is defined as three consecutive early pregnancy losses (empty sac type) or two consecutive fetal losses (loss of fetal heart activity following ultrasound confirmation). The appearance of either of these patient presentations should trigger investigation as maternal thrombophilia may be an underlying cause.

Staffing and training implications

It is vital that only appropriately trained and competent staff perform transabdominal and transvaginal early pregnancy scans. Sonographers, specialist nurses and clinicians should aspire to produce ultrasound reports following standardised Royal College of Radiologists/RCOG documentation. Postgraduate trainees need supervision from their educational supervisor or lead clinician to ensure competency and observation of their skills in examination and scanning as part of their formative assessment of skills.

All recurrent miscarriage clinics should have a designated lead consultant with a special interest in recurrent miscarriage. In addition, all medical and nursing staff should undergo formal training in breaking bad news and in providing emotional and psychological support.

Ideally, all gynaecologists should be able to conduct laparoscopic surgery in the management of ectopic pregnancy. All trainees should be encouraged to complete an Advanced Training Skills Module (ATSM) in early pregnancy and laparoscopic surgery.

Opportunities for specialist training

Training courses are available to specialist trainees as they progress through their careers. It is recommended that trainees complete the modules in intermediate ultrasound in gynaecology and intermediate ultrasound of early pregnancy complications before embarking on the ATSM in acute gynaecology and early pregnancy.

Audit and research issues

As an essential component of clinical governance, all early pregnancy units and recurrent miscarriage clinics should have regular meetings to review clinical guidelines and protocols. This would provide an ideal opportunity to discuss audits and generate research ideas and to discuss recruitment to national or international multicentre trials.

Regular audits should be undertaken and should include patient choice regarding management of miscarriage and ectopic pregnancy and complications associated with the various methods. Units should specifically include the medical and surgical management of ectopic pregnancy and audit the percentage of laparoscopic management of ectopic pregnancy, the rates of ruptured ectopic pregnancies and the incidence of failed diagnosis of ectopic pregnancy.

It is highly recommended to include surveys of patient satisfaction with facilities and counselling to identify areas that need improvement.

Key points

The following key points should be taken into consideration:

○ All women with early pregnancy complications should be evaluated in a dedicated early pregnancy unit.

○ Management of women with early pregnancy complications should be conducted by trained and competent staff.

○ Adequate facilities should exist to perform scans and to measure serum hCG levels.

○ Algorithms should be in place to guide management of spontaneous and recurrent miscarriage, ectopic pregnancy and pregnancy of unknown location.

○ Patients should be offered an informed choice of management options.[7,8]

○ Patients should be furnished with information in non-medical language and supported by written information. There should be access to interpretation services.

○ A quiet room conducive to breaking bad news should be located away from the work area.

○ Bereavement counselling should be offered to all women who suffer a pregnancy loss.

○ Adherence to local and national standards should be audited regularly.

References

1 Lewis G, editor. *The Confidential Enquiry into Maternal and Child Health (CEMACH). Saving mothers' lives: reviewing maternal deaths to make motherhood safer: 2003–2005. The seventh report on Confidential Enquiries into Maternal Deaths in the UK.* London: CEMACH; 2007.

2 Association of Early Pregnancy Units. *Guidelines 2007.* [www.earlypregnancy.org.uk/adminsection/documents/ AEPUGuidelines2007.pdf].

3 Royal College of Obstetricians and Gynaecologists. *Standards for Gynaecology: Report of a Working Party.* London: RCOG Press; 2008. p. 14–19 [www.rcog.org.uk/ womens-health/clinical-guidance/standards-gynaecology].

4 Royal College of Obstetricians and Gynaecologists. *The management of early pregnancy loss.* Green-top Guideline No. 25. London: RCOG; 2006 [www.rcog.org.uk/womens- health/clinical-guidance/management-early-pregnancy-loss- green-top-25].

5 Royal College of Obstetricians and Gynaecologists. *The management of tubal pregnancy.* Green-top Guideline No. 21. London: RCOG; 2004 [www.rcog.org.uk/womens- health/clinical-guidance/management-tubal-pregnancy-21- may-2004].

6 Jauniaux E, Farquharson R G, Christiansen O B, Exalto N. Evidence-based guidelines for the investigation and medical treatment of recurrent miscarriage. *Hum Reprod* 2006;21:2216–22.

7 Trinder J, Brocklehurst P, Porter R, Read M, Vyas S, Smith L. Management of miscarriage: expectant, medical, or surgical? Results of randomised controlled trial (miscarriage treatment (MIST) trial). *BMJ* 2006;332:1235–40.

8 Ankum W M. Management of first trimester miscarriage. *Br J Hosp Med (Lond)* 2008;69:380–3.

2 Epidemiology and aetiology of miscarriage and ectopic pregnancy

Cecilia Bottomley

Introduction

Miscarriage is the most common complication of pregnancy. It rarely causes serious health problems,[1] but it can adversely affect women's social and psychological wellbeing. Ectopic pregnancy is less common than miscarriage, but it remains the leading cause of first-trimester maternal mortality and is associated with significant physical and psychosocial morbidity.

According to the Seventh Report on Confidential Enquiries into Maternal Deaths in the United Kingdom, there are around 1 000 000 pregnancies per year in the UK, with approximately 700 000 deliveries occurring each year.[2] It is estimated that the number of miscarriages per year is at least 200 000 and the number of ectopic pregnancies at least 10 000. The maternal mortality rate in relation to early pregnancy complications in the UK in the 3 years between 2003 and 2005 was 0.47/100 000 maternities for ectopic pregnancy (a total of ten deaths) and 0.05/100 000 maternities for miscarriage (one recorded death).[2] Thus, despite a relatively low mortality rate, the overall impact of these disorders on women's health is significant.

Miscarriage is conventionally quoted to affect one in five pregnancies[3] and ectopic pregnancy to occur in 1/100 gestations; however, establishing the true rate of these early pregnancy complications is challenging owing to the lack of accurate data. Hospital statistics provide information regarding the rate of miscarriage and ectopic pregnancy resulting in hospital admissions. However, the majority of women diagnosed with miscarriage are nowadays managed without admission to hospital. Women with ectopic pregnancies are also increasingly managed as outpatients, either expectantly or by medical treatment with methotrexate. Thus, large proportions of ectopic pregnancy and miscarriage cases are not included in existing hospital admission statistics.

Epidemiological data can also be derived from individual journal publications. These data are discussed in this chapter, although it should be remembered that the rate of pathology described is always dependent on the patient population being studied, the diagnostic criteria used and the accessibility of medical care.

FIGURE 2.1 **Miscarriage and ectopic pregnancies that resulted in an NHS stay: rate/100 deliveries, 1997–98 to 2007–08**

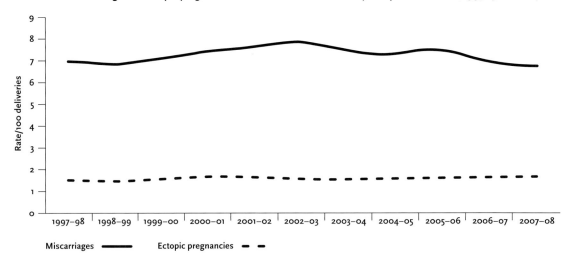

Ectopic pregnancies have remained stable at a rate of approximately 1.6/100 deliveries from 1997–98 to 2007–08. In 2007–08, the miscarriage rate dropped by 0.1 from 6.9/100 deliveries in 2006–07 to 6.8/100 deliveries.

SOURCE: Hospital Episode Statistics, Figure 2, April 2009, with permission.

Miscarriage

Epidemiology

The rate of miscarriage resulting in hospital admission has remained stable over the last 20 years at around seven per 100 deliveries (Figure 2.1). An estimated 25–50% of women experience at least one sporadic miscarriage during their reproductive life.[4]

A study of women followed prospectively for 3 months from the time of conception found a miscarriage rate of 31%.[5] In this group, 41% of miscarriages were biochemical pregnancy failures rather than pregnancies visualised by ultrasound. In another similar study, the pregnancy loss rate was 27% for biochemical pregnancies and 11% for those that were clinically recognised (total miscarriage rate 38%).[6] Regan et al.[7] reported a 12% miscarriage rate in 630 women studied prospectively who underwent ultrasound scan before 8 weeks of gestation.

A prospective community study in a general practice in the UK found that the miscarriage rate was 12% before 20 weeks of gestation.[8] The miscarriage rate at early pregnancy units is higher at 17–46%,[9–11] as would be expected as women often present to these units with clinical symptoms suggestive of early pregnancy failure. Women attending for termination of pregnancy for psychosocial reasons are diagnosed as having delayed miscarriage in 6–11%

FIGURE 2.2 **Miscarriages that resulted in an NHS hospital stay by age: rate/100 deliveries, 2007–08**

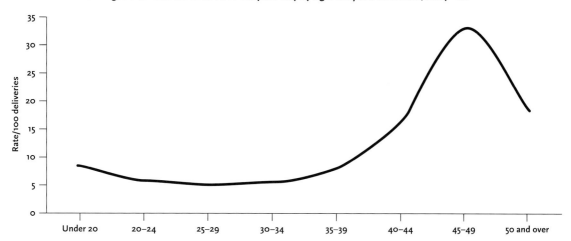

It is extremely difficult to obtain accurate statistics on miscarriages as many remain unreported; however, in 2007–08, of all miscarriages that resulted in a hospital stay, over one-third were within the 45–49-year-old age group.

SOURCE: Hospital Episode Statistics, Figure 4, April 2009, with permission.

of cases.[12–14] At the time of routine first-trimester ultrasound (at 10–13 weeks), delayed miscarriage is found in 3% of women.[15] Overall, it can be seen that the rate of miscarriages decreases with increasing gestational age, as the majority of pregnancy failures occur early. Second-trimester miscarriage is much less common, with a reported incidence of 1–4%.[16]

It is not known whether the overall miscarriage rate is increasing or decreasing with time. However, it is likely that the number of miscarriages diagnosed may be increasing as a result of earlier recognition of pregnancy with easily available highly sensitive urine pregnancy tests and the increasingly routine use of transvaginal ultrasonography in early pregnancy units.

Risk factors

Maternal age
Hospital admission data show variations in miscarriage rates with age (Figure 2.2). The link between maternal age and increased miscarriage rate, especially after the age of 35 years, is well established.[17] Women less than 35 years of age have a 9–12% clinical miscarriage rate. However, the rate is greater than 45% in women over the age of 40 years. This relates predominantly to the increased rate of trisomies with maternal age, as discussed further in the aetiology section of this chapter.

Previous obstetric history

One study reported an overall miscarriage rate of 12%; however, women whose previous pregnancies had all been unsuccessful had a 24% miscarriage rate, whereas primigravid or parous women had a miscarriage rate of 4–5%.[7]

Recurrent miscarriage, defined as three or more consecutive miscarriages, affects 1–5% of couples.[4,18] This figure is higher than would be expected considering the risk of sporadic miscarriage, hence the tradition of investigating women who have had three consecutive losses for the specific causes of pregnancy failure rather than simply assuming recurrent sporadic loss.

Lifestyle and nutrition

Smoking is associated with an increased risk of miscarriage,[19,20] as is regular or high alcohol consumption.[21] Low prepregnancy body mass index is also associated with a higher rate of early pregnancy loss.[21]

Aetiology

First-trimester miscarriage

The majority of miscarriages are attributable to chromosomal abnormalities. Further aetiological factors that are associated with first-trimester miscarriage include teratogenic drugs (see chapter 8), maternal medical conditions and maternal uterine abnormalities.[16]

CHROMOSOMAL ABNORMALITIES

As genetic testing techniques have developed, the proportion of miscarriages that can be attributed to chromosomal abnormalities has increased from 50% using karyotyping of cultured placental tissue[22] to more than 70% using comparative genomic hybridisation.[23] The abnormalities are approximately 70% trisomies, 20% triploidies and 10% monosomy X. The most common trisomies associated with miscarriage are 6, 21 and 22. The prevalence of these aneuploidies increases with maternal age, owing to the age-related error at first meiotic divison. This age-related change is demonstrated in Figure 2.3, which also shows that the rate of non-trisomic and euploid miscarriage does not vary significantly with age.[24]

The rate of chromosomal abnormalities causing miscarriage decreases with increasing gestational age.[4] It has been estimated that 50–80% of first-trimester losses are associated with a chromosomal abnormality, whereas in the second and third trimesters the proportion of pregnancy losses caused by a chromosomal abnormality is 15% and 5%, respectively.

FIGURE 2.3 **Graph demonstrating that the increase in the incidence of miscarriage with maternal age relates predominantly to an increase in trisomy, as the rate of non-trisomic miscarriage remains relatively constant**

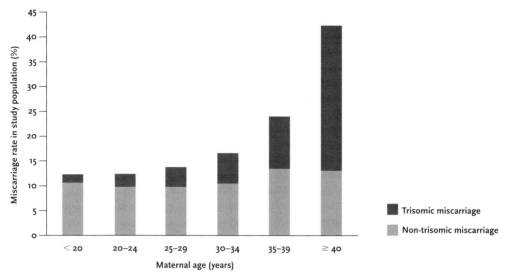

SOURCE: Hassold and Chiu, 1985, with permission.[24]

PARENTAL STRUCTURAL CHROMOSOMAL ABNORMALITY

In 3–5% of couples with a history of recurrent miscarriage, one parent is affected by a structural chromosomal abnormality. Balanced translocation, which occurs in 1/625 of the adult population,[25] accounts for two-thirds of such abnormalities and more commonly affects the mother than the father.[26] The effect of such a translocation depends on the specific duplicated or deleted sequences, with affected carriers being more likely to miscarry.

MATERNAL MEDICAL CONDITIONS

There is a higher miscarriage rate among women with diabetes compared with women without diabetes, especially if prepregnancy glucose control is poor.[27] However, the rate of miscarriage in women with diabetes was reported in one study to be only 13.5%.[28]

Thyroid disease increases the miscarriage rate if it is undiagnosed or poorly controlled. There is also increasing interest in the role of antithyroid antibodies in miscarriage. The prevalence of these antibodies increases with maternal age and women positive for antithyroid antibodies have a two- to four-fold greater risk of first-trimester miscarriage, even when they appear euthyroid. It is not clear whether this is because the presence of antibodies is a marker for a generalised autoimmune disease or because these women have subtle disturbances in their thyroid function.[29]

Women with systemic lupus erythematosus have been shown to have an increased miscarriage rate of 20%.[30] The presence of antiphosholipid antibodies (found in 1–3% of the healthy fertile population), whether primary or secondary to another condition such as systemic lupus, is associated with recurrent miscarriage.[31] Rather than causing miscarriage through a prothrombotic effect, it is now thought that the pathophysiology involves inflammation at the maternal–fetal interface and deficient placentation with reduced trophoblast invasion and poor spiral artery transformation.[32]

MATERNAL UTERINE ANOMALIES

Congenital uterine abnormalities have been examined for their role in miscarriage. The rate of congenital anomalies in women with recurrent miscarriage is greater than in control populations (24% versus 5%).[33] More than 90% of such abnormalities are either subseptate or arcuate uteri. Major anomalies are found in 2–7% of women with recurrent miscarriage compared with 1.7–2.3% of women with normal reproductive outcome.[33,34] It is likely that a relatively avascular septum is unable to provide an adequate blood supply or to adapt for trophoblast invasion of the implanting embryo.

LUTEAL PHASE DEFECT

It has been postulated that in some women who miscarry there is a luteal phase defect occurring as a result of a gonadotrophin-releasing hormone, luteinising hormone or endometrial receptor defect. There are no validated diagnostic criteria for such a diagnosis and, although progesterone supplementation has been used to overcome this possible deficiency, the effectiveness of such treatment has never been confirmed.

Second-trimester miscarriage

The spectrum of pathology associated with second-trimester miscarriage is different from that of first-trimester miscarriage. (Early embryonic demise that occurs before 12 weeks of gestation but where the embryo remains retained within the uterus into the second trimester should be classified as first-trimester loss.) Causes of second-trimester miscarriage include infection (chorioamnionitis or maternal systemic infection), cervical weakness, structural uterine abnormalities and thrombophilia. Genetic causes may still play a role in second-trimester miscarriage, although where a genetic abnormality is involved (estimated to occur in 15% of cases) the abnormality tends to be one that is occasionally seen in term deliveries (trisomies 13, 18 and 21, monosomy X and sex chromosome polysomies) or that involves a gene mutation or deletion.[35]

TABLE 2.1 **Incidence of ectopic pregnancy in different countries**

Country	Rate
UK[2]	11/1000
Norway[44]	15/1000
Australia[45]	16/1000
USA[46]	20/1000
Central Africa[36]	8/1000

Ectopic pregnancy

Epidemiology

Hospital admission statistics suggest that the rate of ectopic pregnancy resulting in hospital admission is 1.5/100 deliveries (1.5%) and that this rate is stable (Figure 2.1). Reported incidences in other countries are shown in Table 2.1. However, these rates rely on very different methodologies and caution should be exercised in the interpretation of these reports.

The mortality rate from ectopic pregnancy in the UK is around 0.47/100 000 maternities. This has remained fairly constant over the last 20 years. In African developing countries it is reported as 1–3%, ten times higher than that reported in industrialised countries.[36]

In early pregnancy units (in the UK) the rate of ectopic pregnancy is around 2–3%,[37] reflecting the fact that women presenting to an early pregnancy unit are already at an inherently higher risk of poor outcome.

Risk factors

Maternal associations with ectopic pregnancy include age, past history of sexually transmitted infection, infertility, smoking, intrauterine contraception, tubal infection, pelvic surgery and in vitro fertilisation (IVF). The important association between age and ectopic pregnancy diagnosis is also demonstrated in UK hospital admission statistics (Figure 2.4). Appendicectomy does not increase the risk of ectopic pregnancy unless the appendix has ruptured. One meta-analysis has categorised the known risk factors into those that confer a strongly or mildly increased risk of ectopic pregnancy:[38]

FIGURE 2.4 **Ectopic pregnancies that resulted in an NHS stay by age: rate/100 deliveries in an NHS hospital, England, 2006–07**

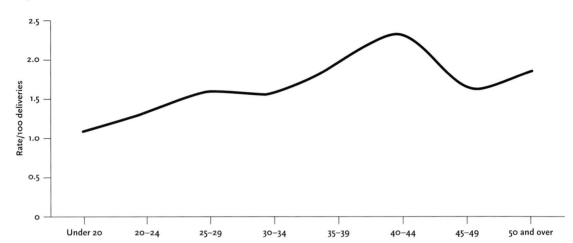

The highest rate of ectopic pregnancies occurred in the 40–44-year-old age group (2.3/100 deliveries) and the lowest was in the under 20 years of age group (1.1/100 deliveries).

SOURCE: Hospital Episode Statistics, Figure 3, September 2008, with permission.

- Strongly increased risk:
  - previous ectopic pregnancy
  - previous tubal surgery
  - documented tubal pathology
  - in utero diethylstilbestrol exposure.

- Moderately increased risk:
  - previous genital infections (pelvic inflammatory disease, chlamydia, gonorrhoea)
  - infertility
  - lifetime number of sexual partners greater than one.

A large French study[39] of all ectopic pregnancies diagnosed in one region showed the most important risk factors to be history of infection and smoking. The other risk factors were maternal age, past history of miscarriage, history of medical (but not surgical) termination of pregnancy, history of infertility and previous use of an intrauterine contraceptive device. The total attributable risk of ectopic pregnancy for known risk factors was 0.76: that is, 24% of women with a diagnosis of ectopic pregnancy had no known risk factors. Absolute risks for ectopic pregnancy in some conditions have also been calculated (Table 2.2). It is important to remember that although factors such as

TABLE 2.2 **Risk factors for ectopic pregnancy**

Risk factor	Risk of ectopic pregnancy (%)
After IVF [47]	4
After sterilisation [48]	0.7*
After PID [49]	10
After previous ectopic pregnancy [50]	8–18

*Within 10 years of the procedure. IVF = in vitro fertilisation | PID = pelvic inflammatory disease.

previous ectopic pregnancy, documented tubal pathology or IVF confer the highest risk of ectopic pregnancy, many women with ectopic pregnancies will not have such risk factors. The risk factors that apply to a larger number of women (such as increased maternal age, smoking and a history of infertility) in fact have a higher overall impact on the incidence of ectopic pregnancy. This is demonstrated in Table 2.3, which shows that the highest attributable risk for ectopic pregnancy is smoking.[39]

The increase in the rate of smoking, use of assisted conception techniques, chlamydia infections and tubal pathology would all be expected to result in an increase in the incidence of ectopic pregnancy. In addition, it would be

TABLE 2.3 **Adjusted attributable risk of the main risk factors for ectopic pregnancy according to the register of the Auvergne region, France, 1993–2000** [39]

Variables	Adjusted attributable risk
Woman's age	0.14
Past or current smoking	0.35
Prior spontaneous miscarriage(s)	0.07
Prior termination of pregnancy	0.03
Appendicectomy	0.02
Prior sexually transmitted diseases	0.18
Prior tubal surgery	0.18
Prior sexually transmitted diseases and tubal surgery	0.33
Previous use of oral contraceptive*	0.08
Previous use of intrauterine device	0.05
History of infertility	0.18
Total	**0.76**

*Attributable risk for not using oral contraceptive.

expected that the advent and wide use of high-resolution ultrasound machines would result in more ectopic pregnancies being diagnosed. Indeed, there is some evidence that the rates did increase during the 1980s and 1990s.[40] However, as shown in Figure 2.1, the rate of ectopic pregnancy in the UK seems to have been stable over the last 20 years and the mortality rate of 0.4 deaths per 1000 ectopic pregnancies has also remained static.[2]

Aetiology

The many associations with ectopic pregnancy have been described above. However, the pathophysiology of tubal implantation is not clear. The quality of the fertilised ovum is a possible contributory factor. A suggestion that ectopic pregnancies are more likely to be chromosomally abnormal has not been properly validated.[41,42] A possible effect of the male partner in the aetiology of ectopic pregnancy has also not been confirmed.[43] Impaired migration of the fertilised ovum in the fallopian tube appears to be the main factor in most cases. This may be due to physical damage to the tube from infection or previous surgery. Smoking may affect all aspects of reproduction including ovulation, fertilisation, transport of the fertilised ovum and implantation.

Conclusion

The rate of miscarriage is largely determined by the characteristics of the population being studied, and can range from 3% to 41%. Clinically recognised pregnancies are miscarried in 12–30% of cases. The large majority of miscarriages are attributable to sporadic chromosomal abnormalities, leading to a good prognosis for future pregnancies. Causes such as poorly controlled diabetes, thyroid disease or autoantibody conditions are less common, although potentially treatable.

Ectopic pregnancy occurs in around 1% of the general population and in 2–3% of the early pregnancy population. Strong associations have been found between ectopic pregnancy and IVF, previous pelvic infection or surgery. However, history of infertility, advancing maternal age and smoking are equally important factors. The pathophysiology of ectopic pregnancy remains unclear.

References

1 Trinder J, Brocklehurst P, Porter R, Read M, Vyas S, Smith L. Management of miscarriage: expectant, medical, or surgical? Results of randomised controlled trial (miscarriage treatment (MIST) trial). *BMJ* 2006;332:1235–40.

2 Lewis G, editor. *The Confidential Enquiry into Maternal and Child Health (CEMACH). Saving mothers' lives: reviewing maternal deaths to make motherhood safer: 2003–2005. The seventh report on Confidential Enquiries into Maternal Deaths in the UK*. London: CEMACH; 2007.

3 Savitz D A, Hertz-Picciotto I, Poole C, Olshan A F. Epidemiologic measures of the course and outcome of pregnancy. *Epidemiol Rev* 2002;24:91–101.

4 Stephenson M, Kutteh W. Evaluation and management of recurrent early pregnancy loss. *Clin Obstet Gynecol* 2007;50:132–45.

5 Zinaman M J, Clegg D E, Brown C C, O'Connor J, Selevan S G. Estimates of human fertility and pregnancy loss. *Fertil Steril* 1996;65:503–9.

6 Ellish N J, Saboda K, O'Connor J O, Nasca P C, Stanek E J, Boyle C. A prospective study of early pregnancy loss. *Hum Reprod* 1996;11:406–12.

7 Regan L, Braude P R, Trembath P L. Influence of past reproductive performance on risk of spontaneous abortion. *BMJ* 1989;299:541–5.

8 Everett C. Incidence and outcome of bleeding before the 20th week of pregnancy: prospective study from general practice. *BMJ* 1997;315:32–4.

9 Bigrigg M A, Read M D. Management of women referred to early pregnancy assessment unit: care and cost effectiveness. *BMJ* 1991;302:577–9.

10 Shillito J, Walker J J. Early pregnancy assessment units. *Br J Hosp Med* 1997;58:505–9.

11 Schauberger C W, Mathiason M A, Rooney B L. Ultrasound assessment of first-trimester bleeding. *Obstet Gynecol* 2005;105:333–8.

12 Acharya G, Morgan H, Paramanantham L, Fernando R. A randomized controlled trial comparing surgical termination of pregnancy with and without continuous ultrasound guidance. *Eur J Obstet Gynecol Reprod Biol* 2004;114:69–74.

13 McGalliard C, Gaudoin M. Routine ultrasound for pregnancy termination requests increases women's choice and reduces inappropriate treatments. *BJOG* 2004;111:79–82.

14 Sinha P, Pradhan A, Chowdhury V. Value of routine transvaginal ultrasound scan in women requesting early termination of pregnancy. *J Obstet Gynaecol* 2004;24:426–8.

15 Pandya P P, Snijders R J, Psara N, Hilbert L, Nicolaides K H. The prevalence of non-viable pregnancy at 10–13 weeks of gestation. *Ultrasound Obstet Gynecol* 1996;7:170–3.

16 Regan L, Rai R. Epidemiology and the medical causes of miscarriage. *Baillieres Best Pract Res Clin Obstet Gynaecol* 2000;14:839–54.

17 Nybo Andersen A M, Wohlfahrt J, Christens P, Olsen J, Melbye M. Maternal age and fetal loss: population based register linkage study. *BMJ* 2000;320:1708–12.

18 Rai R, Regan L. Recurrent miscarriage. *Lancet* 2006;368:601–11.

19 Shiverick K T, Salafia C. Cigarette smoking and pregnancy I: ovarian, uterine and placental effects. *Placenta* 1990;20:265–72.

20 Waylen A L, Metwally M, Jones G L, Wilkinson A J, Ledger W L. Effects of cigarette smoking upon clinical outcomes of assisted reproduction: a meta-analysis. *Hum Reprod Update* 2009;15:31–44.

21 Maconochie N, Doyle P, Prior S, Simmons R. Risk factors for first trimester miscarriage: results from a UK-population-based case–control study. *BJOG* 2007;114:170–86.

22 Hassold T, Chen N, Funkhouser J, Jooss T, Manuel B, Matsuura J, et al. A cytogenetic study of 1000 spontaneous abortions. *Ann Hum Genet* 1980;44:151–78.

23 Fritz B, Hallermann C, Olert J, Fuchs B, Bruns M, Aslan M, et al. Cytogenetic analyses of culture failures by comparative genomic hybridisation (CGH) – re-evaluation of chromosome aberration rates in early spontaneous abortions. *Eur J Hum Genet* 2001;9:539–47.

24 Hassold T, Chiu D. Maternal age-specific rates of numerical chromosome abnormalities with special reference to trisomy. *Hum Genet* 1985;70:11–7.

25 Van Dyke D L, Weiss L, Roberson J R, Babu V R. The frequency and mutation rate of balanced autosomal rearrangements in man estimated from prenatal genetic studies for advanced maternal age. *Am J Hum Genet* 1983;35:301–8.

26 Goddijn M, Joosten J H, Knegt A C, van derVeen F, Franssen M T, Bonsel GJ, et al. Clinical relevance of diagnosing structural chromosome abnormalities in couples with repeated miscarriage. *Hum Reprod* 2004;19:1013–7.

27 Galindo A, Burguillo AG, Azriel S, Fuente Pde L. Outcome of fetuses in women with pregestational diabetes mellitus. *J Perinat Med* 2006;34:323–31.

28 Pearson D, Kernaghan D, Lee R, Penney G; Scottish Diabetes in Pregnancy Study Group. The relationship between pre-pregnancy care and early pregnancy loss, major congenital anomaly or perinatal death in type I diabetes mellitus. *BJOG* 2007;114:104–7.

29 Glinoer D. The systematic screening and management of hypothyroidism and hyperthyroidism during pregnancy. *Trends Endocrinol Metab* 1998;10:403–11.

30 Molad Y, Borkowski T, Monselise A, Ben-Haroush A, Sulkes J, Hod M, et al. Maternal and fetal outcome of lupus pregnancy: a prospective study of 29 pregnancies. *Lupus* 2005;14:145–51.

31 Rai RS, Clifford K, Cohen H, Regan L. High prospective fetal loss rate in untreated pregnancies of women with recurrent miscarriage and antiphospholipid antibodies. *Hum Reprod* 1995;10:3301–4.

32 Abrahams V M. Mechanisms of antiphospholipid antibody-associated pregnancy complications. *Thromb Res* 2009;124:521–5.

33 Salim R, Regan L, Woelfer B, Backos M, Jurkovic D. A comparative study of the morphology of congenital uterine anomalies in women with and without a history of recurrent first trimester miscarriage. *Hum Reprod* 2003;18:162–6.

34 Jurkovic D, Gruboeck K, Tailor A, Nicolaides K H. Ultrasound screening for congenital uterine anomalies. *Br J Obstet Gynaecol* 1997;104:1320–1.

35 Simpson J L. Causes of fetal wastage. *Clin Obstet Gynecol* 2007;50:10–30.

36 Goyaux N, Leke R, Keita N, Thonneau P. Ectopic pregnancy in African developing countries. *Acta Obstet Gynecol Scand* 2003;82:305–12.

37 Kirk E, Condous G, Haider Z, Lu C, Van Huffel S, Timmerman D, et al. The practical application of a mathematical model to predict the outcome of pregnancies of unknown location. *Ultrasound Obstet Gynecol* 2006;27:311–5.

38 Ankum W M, Mol B W, Van der Veen F, Bossuyt P M. Risk factors for ectopic pregnancy: a meta-analysis. *Fertil Steril* 1996;65:1093–9.

39 Bouyer J, Coste J, Shojaei T, Pouly J L, Fernandez H, Gerbaud L, et al. Risk factors for ectopic pregnancy: a comprehensive analysis based on a large case-control, population-based study in France. *Am J Epidemiol* 2003;157:185–94.

40 Chow W H, Daling J R, Cates W Jr, Greenberg R S. Epidemiology of ectopic pregnancy. *Epidemiol Rev* 1987;9:70–94.

41 Coste J, Fernandez H, Joyé N, Benifla J, Girard S, Marpeau L, et al. Role of chromosome abnormalities in ectopic pregnancy. *Fertil Steril* 2000;74:1259–60.

42 Goddijn M, van der Veen F, Schuring-Blom GH, Ankum W M, Leschot N J. Cytogenetic characteristics of ectopic pregnancy. *Hum Reprod* 1996;11:2769–71.

43 Warnes G M, Petrucco O M, Seamark R F, Lancaster P A. Is the male involved in the aetiology of ectopic pregnancy? *Hum Reprod* 1998;13:3505–10.

44 Bakken I J, Skjeldestad F E. Reduced number of extrauterine pregnancies – increased fertility of women during the 1990s? *Tidsskr Nor Laegeforen* 2003;123:3011–4.

45 Boufous S, Quartararo M, Mohsin M, Parker J. Trends in the incidence of ectopic pregnancy in New South Wales between 1990–1998. *Aust N Z J Obstet Gynaecol* 2001;41:436–8.

46 From the Centers for Disease Control and Prevention. Ectopic pregnancy—United States, 1990–1992. *JAMA* 1995;273:533.

47 Fernandez H, Gervaise A. Ectopic pregnancies after infertility treatment: modern diagnosis and therapeutic strategy. *Hum Reprod Update* 2004;10:503–13.

48 Peterson H B, Xia Z, Hughes J M, Wilcox L S, Tylor LR, Trussell J. The risk of ectopic pregnancy after tubal sterilization. U.S. Collaborative Review of Sterilization Working Group. *N Engl J Med* 1997;336:762–7.

49 Tay J I, Moore J, Walker J J. Ectopic pregnancy. *BMJ* 2000;320:916–9.

50 Silva P, Schaper A, Rooney B. Reproductive outcome after 143 laparoscopic procedures for ectopic pregnancy. *Obstet Gyencol* 1993;81:710–5.

3 Diagnosis of miscarriage

Michelle Swer and Davor Jurkovic

Introduction

Miscarriage is the most common complication in early pregnancy. It occurs in 15% of clinically recognised pregnancies[1] and accounts for 50 000 inpatient hospital admissions each year in the UK.[2] In recent years early pregnancy units have been designed to improve the quality of service in the diagnosis of early pregnancy complications and provide rapid and accessible care.

The prevalence of miscarriage in early pregnancy units varies from 17% to 46%.[3,4] The management of women with suspected or confirmed miscarriage is the main task for medical professionals with an interest in providing early pregnancy care. The introduction of ultrasound into routine clinical practice has greatly improved the diagnosis and management of early pregnancy complications. However, easier access to dedicated early pregnancy services has also led to an increasing number of women seeking advice at early gestations. The main challenge in the provision of modern early pregnancy care is balancing the need for sympathetic and individualised care of women who have suffered early pregnancy loss with the need to manage a large number of patients on a routine daily basis.

Terminology

A miscarriage can be defined as a pregnancy failure occurring before the completion of 24 weeks of gestation, which is the current threshold for fetal viability. Miscarriages are classified as early (less than 12 weeks of gestation) or late (from 12 to 24 weeks of gestation). The risk of miscarriage decreases with increasing gestational age and late miscarriages occur in only 1–4% of cases (Figure 3.1). Recurrent miscarriage is the occurrence of three or more consecutive miscarriages, and affects 1% of all women of reproductive age.

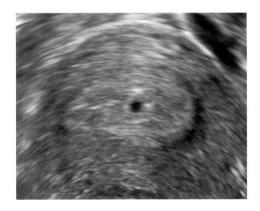

FIGURE 3.1 **A longitudinal section through the uterus showing a normal intrauterine pregnancy at 4 weeks of gestation**

A variety of terms have been used to describe the types of miscarriage. In 2005, the European Society for Human Reproduction and Embryology's Special Interest Group in Early Pregnancy published a revised nomenclature for the various early pregnancy events.[5] Although these terms are accepted as standardised terminology by the RCOG in the UK, they have not been universally adopted.

Diagnosis of miscarriage on clinical examination

Miscarriage is suspected in a woman who presents with vaginal bleeding and/ or loss of pregnancy symptoms. Traditionally, miscarriage was classified as threatened, inevitable or complete, with the type of miscarriage identified on the basis of history and findings on speculum examination. A threatened miscarriage was identified by a history of vaginal bleeding and a closed cervical os, with a presumed continuing intrauterine pregnancy. A diagnosis of inevitable miscarriage was made by speculum examination findings of products of conception and/or an open cervical os. These two terms are less often used in modern clinical practice. A complete miscarriage was diagnosed in women who had passed products of conception and in whom bleeding had stopped spontaneously.

Wieringa-de Waard et al.[6] carried out a prospective study to determine the diagnostic value of history taking and physical examination in first-trimester bleeding. The results showed that the diagnosis of miscarriage based on clinical signs and symptoms is inaccurate in more than 50% of cases.[6] This proves that a clinical diagnosis of miscarriage is unreliable and that pelvic examination, including speculum examination, should be mainly used in women who present with heavy bleeding and who are haemodynamically unstable. In such instances a speculum examination can detect retained products protruding through the cervix and facilitate their removal. In women who present with mild symptoms, an ultrasound scan is more helpful than clinical examination and should be used as a primary test to assess the viability of the pregnancy.

Ultrasound findings

Ultrasound has become the mainstay in the diagnosis of miscarriage and is offered routinely to any woman in whom miscarriage is suspected. Traditionally, early pregnancy scans were carried out transabdominally; however, 42% of women examined transabdominally also required a transvaginal scan owing to poor views because of an underfilled bladder or the inconclusive nature of the scan.[3] In modern practice transvaginal ultrasonography has become the accepted standard for the examination of women with suspected early pregnancy complications. It provides much clearer images, can be used at earlier gestations and does not require a full bladder.

The aim of ultrasound in early pregnancy complications is two-fold:

- diagnosis of early pregnancy failure

- prediction of outcome in potentially viable pregnancies.

With the use of ultrasound parameters, miscarriage can now be broadly classified into three groups: early embryonic demise, incomplete miscarriage and complete miscarriage. It is important to have strict diagnostic criteria in place to avoid misdiagnosis. This is especially important in women who are unsure of their dates, have irregular cycles, conceived while on contraception or have had fewer than three menstrual periods since their last pregnancy.

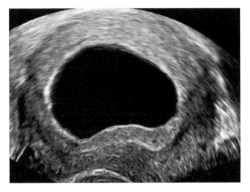

FIGURE 3.2 **A large gestational sac measuring 33 mm in the mean diameter with no evidence of a yolk sac or an embryo**

These findings are conclusive of an early embryonic demise.

Diagnosis of miscarriage

Early embryonic demise

In a normal early pregnancy the size of the gestational sac may be used to estimate gestational age. The sac usually becomes visible at 4[+3] weeks of gestation and grows approximately 1 mm per day during the first trimester. An embryo can be seen within a gestational sac, which can be as small as 10 mm. A large gestational sac with the absence of an embryo is a well-established indicator of early embryonic demise. However, there is no consensus as to the optimal cut-off size of the gestational sac for establishing a miscarriage. Different studies have shown cut-off points of 16 mm, 17 mm or 18 mm as possible predictors of non-viability;[7-9] however, Elson et al. have shown that normal pregnancies may occasionally present with a gestational sac greater than 18 mm with no visible embryo on the initial scan (Figure 3.2).[10]

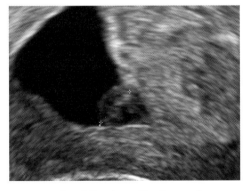

FIGURE 3.3 **A gestational sac with a 6 mm embryo with no visible cardiac activity on B-mode examination in a woman who suffered a miscarriage**

TABLE 3.1 **Ultrasound criteria for the diagnosis of early embryonic demise**

Ultrasound findings	Action
Gestational sac >20 mm with no embryo or yolk sac	Repeat scan in 1 week
Crown–rump length >10 mm with no heart action	Repeat scan in 1 week
Gestational sac <15 mm or crown–rump length <10 mm	Repeat scan in 2 weeks

SOURCE: Hatley W, Case J, Campbell S. Establishing the death of an embryo by ultrasound: report of a public enquiry with recommendations. *Ultrasound Obstet Gynecol* 1995;5:353–7.

Cardiac activity is not detectable on transabdominal scan in one-third of normal embryos with a crown–rump length (CRL) of less than 5 mm. However, there is a 91% miscarriage rate when cardiac activity is not visible on transvaginal scan in embryos measuring less than 5 mm.[11] Some studies have diagnosed miscarriage reliably, both transvaginally and transabdominally, with embryos measuring ≥4 mm (Figure 3.3).[12]

These results illustrate the difficulties that are often encountered when the diagnosis of miscarriage is based on negative findings rather than on identification of a specific morphological abnormality. Whichever cut-off points are used to make the diagnosis of miscarriage, it is inevitable that occasionally a very small live embryo will be missed on examination. These errors may occur because of difficulties in visualising the uterus, presence of uterine pathology such as fibroids, operator inexperience or poor-quality ultrasound equipment.

In response to widely publicised cases of normal pregnancies being misdiagnosed as miscarriages, a Joint Working Party of the Royal College of Radiologists and the RCOG was formed to produce guidelines for preventing similar problems occurring in the future. The working party designed guidelines for ultrasound diagnosis of early embryonic demise, which are shown in Table 3.1.[13,14] The guidelines stipulate that the diagnosis of early embryonic demise cannot be made on the first scan and that follow-up is essential even if the findings are highly suggestive of an abnormal pregnancy. The diagnosis of miscarriage should always be made after a follow-up scan that fails to demonstrate the presence of a live embryo.

These criteria have been criticised for being too cautious, delaying the diagnosis of early embryonic demise and increasing maternal anxiety. However, these guidelines are suitable for units where the examinations are performed by less experienced operators without senior supervision and support. They minimise the risk of diagnostic error and facilitate the use of expectant management of miscarriage by delaying the diagnosis for 1 or 2 weeks.

In specialised units with a high level of expertise in ultrasound, a conclusive diagnosis of early embryonic demise can be made on a first visit if one or more of the following parameters is noted on ultrasound:

- the presence of a gestational sac with a mean diameter >20 mm with no visible embryo

- the presence of an embryo with a CRL ≤5 mm with no cardiac activity

- the presence of a yolk sac and amniotic sac with an embryonic pole with no cardiac activity (Figure 3.4).

To minimise the risk of error, in each case the diagnosis should be confirmed by at least one additional independent operator. The advice of senior colleagues should always be sought if there is any uncertainly about the diagnosis, the uterus is abnormal or the ultrasound views are suboptimal.

Incomplete miscarriage

An incomplete miscarriage is defined by the presence of retained products without a well-defined gestational sac. The ultrasound diagnosis of an incomplete miscarriage is more difficult to define and there is no consensus regarding the best diagnostic criteria. The description of retained products varies from heterogeneous irregular echoes in the midline of the uterine cavity[15] to a well-defined area of hyperechoic tissue within the uterine cavity in comparison with blood clots, which are poorly outlined (Figure 3.5).[16] Colour Doppler assessment can be used to facilitate differential diagnosis between retained products and blood clots within the uterine cavity. Retained products are usually well perfused, while no Doppler signals are found originating from blood clots (Figure 3.6).

Endometrial thickness (measured as the anteroposterior diameter of the uterine cavity) has been used by some to aid in the diagnosis of incomplete miscarriage. A number of studies have looked at various cut-off levels, whose values have ranged from 5 mm to 15 mm.[17–20] However, recent studies have shown that

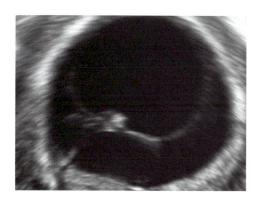

FIGURE 3.4 **A gestational sac containing an amniotic membrane**

These findings are conclusive of a miscarriage.

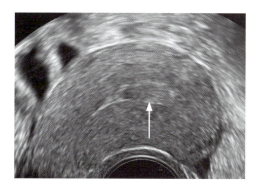

FIGURE 3.5 **A small amount of well-defined retained products of conception (arrow) in a case of incomplete miscarriage**

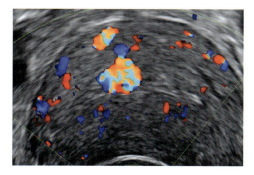

FIGURE 3.6 **On Doppler examination the tissue is highly vascular, which facilitates the diagnosis of retained products of conception**

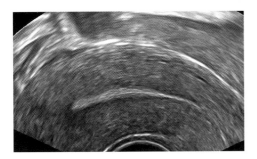

FIGURE 3.7 **An empty uterine cavity in a woman following a complete miscarriage**

A conclusive diagnosis of early embryonic demise was made on the previous scan.

none of the cut-off measurements is accurate enough to diagnose the presence of chorionic villi within the uterine cavity.[21] A subjective assessment of the retained tissue is therefore more helpful in diagnosis than any cut-off measurements.

The main objective in diagnosing an incomplete miscarriage is to clarify whether retained trophoblastic tissue is the likely cause of persistent bleeding in women with a history of recent miscarriage. Those women with evidence of incomplete miscarriage may opt for dilatation and curettage to stop the bleeding and facilitate recovery after miscarriage. There is no correlation between the amount of retained tissue and clinical symptoms. Therefore, surgery should be offered to any woman with persistent bleeding, even if the amount of retained products is very small.

Complete miscarriage

The diagnosis of complete miscarriage is made in women in whom ultrasound examination fails to identify any pregnancy tissue within the uterine cavity. This diagnosis can be made with confidence only in women who had clear evidence of an intrauterine pregnancy on a previous ultrasound examination. If no scan has previously been performed, the pregnancy should be described as a 'pregnancy of unknown location' and should be followed up with biochemical markers (Figure 3.7). This policy ensures that small, slowly developing ectopic pregnancies that are not detectable on the initial scan are not missed.

Prediction of miscarriage

The presence of an embryonic heart rate at the time of the initial ultrasound scan does not always denote a normal pregnancy. A number of other morphological features have to be assessed to estimate the likelihood of favourable pregnancy outcome. An awareness of these parameters will enable appropriate counselling to be given to women regarding the likelihood of a continuing viable pregnancy. However, it is important to be mindful that these findings are not specific enough to make a conclusive diagnosis of pregnancy failure and usually further scans are necessary to monitor the progress of pregnancy.

FIGURE 3.8 **Risk of miscarriage in relation to maternal age**

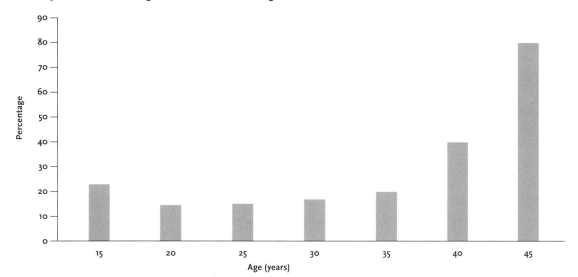

SOURCE: Modified from Nyboe Andresen et al., *BMJ*, 2000,[2] with permission.

Demographic characteristics

Maternal age at conception, previous miscarriages and multigravidity are all known risk factors for miscarriage. Maternal age is a strong and independent risk factor, irrespective of the woman's reproductive history. The risk of miscarriage increases from 8.9% at 22 years of age to 74.7% at 45 years of age or more (Figure 3.8).[22] As an increasing number of women are delaying childbirth for social reasons, this information should be included when counselling women about their chances of successful reproduction.

Gestational sac

A normal sac is round or ovoid in shape, contains anechoic fluid and is surrounded by a thick layer of trophoblast. The shape, position and trophoblastic reaction of the gestational sac can be predictive of early pregnancy failure.[8] A sac with an irregular or angular appearance is associated with an increased risk of miscarriage. However, care should be taken to avoid misinterpreting the presence of a small amount of fluid within the uterine cavity ('pseudo-sac') as an irregular gestational sac. The low position of the gestational sac within the uterine cavity and the finding of a thin trophoblastic shell are additional subjective findings that indicate an increased risk of miscarriage (Figure 3.9).

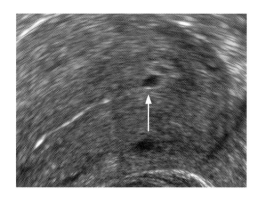

FIGURE 3.9 **A small amount of fluid at the uterine fundus (arrow), resembling a gestational sac, in a woman with a history of vaginal bleeding in early pregnancy**

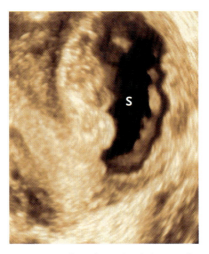

FIGURE 3.10 **Three-dimensional ultrasound image of an irregular gestational sac (S) with no visible embryo**

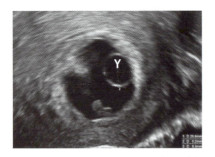

FIGURE 3.11 **An abnormally large yolk sac (Y) in a women who suffered a miscarriage 7 days later**

The use of three-dimensional ultrasound to assess the volume of the gestational sac has not been beneficial in the diagnosis of miscarriage. However, further work is needed to assess whether abnormal gestational sac volume could be used to estimate the risk of miscarriage in pregnancies with a visible embryonic heart rate (Figure 3.10).[23]

Yolk sac

In normal pregnancies, the yolk sac can be identified by the time the mean diameter of the gestational sac measures ≥8 mm.[24] The yolk sac diameter shows a uniform slow growth from 7 to 9 weeks of gestation to a mean size of 4.9 mm, after which it regresses.[25]

A variation from this growth pattern is associated with an abnormal pregnancy outcome. Studies have shown that a yolk sac diameter greater than 5.6 mm in a pregnancy with a duration of less than 10 weeks is strongly associated with a poor pregnancy outcome.[26] This was also noted in a recent study in which, in a pregnancy with a yolk sac diameter above the 95th percentile, miscarriage occurred 10 days later (Figure 3.11).[27] However, this study did not find any significant association between yolk sac size and fetal loss. There have been associations between poor pregnancy outcome and the absence of a yolk sac in the presence of an embryo or a gestational sac measuring more than 8 mm.[24,26] In cases where the pregnancy progresses beyond the first trimester, a detailed fetal anomaly scan is recommended before 20 weeks of gestation.

Amniotic sac

The amniotic membrane becomes visible by 7 weeks of gestation, thus defining the amniotic cavity and the chorionic cavity. The mean diameter of the amniotic cavity is closely correlated to the CRL.[28] Studies have shown that a disproportionately large amniotic cavity relative to the CRL can be a predictor of miscarriage.[29]

Crown–rump length

Measurement of the CRL is used to confirm the gestational age of the pregnancy. In normal pregnancies, CRL can sometimes appear small for gestational age owing to late ovulation or inaccuracies in recording the date of the last menstrual period. However, studies have shown that in a woman with certain menstrual dates, a smaller than expected CRL at the initial scan is a powerful indicator of increased risk of miscarriage even in the presence of normal embryonic cardiac activity.[30,31] A study in 2008 showed that the CRL was at least two standard deviations below the expected size in two-thirds of pregnancies that ended in miscarriage.[31] It is therefore appropriate to consider arranging follow-up for women with initial scan findings of smaller than expected CRL to avoid providing false reassurance.

Embryonic heart rate

The normal first-trimester embryonic heart rate rises from an average of 100 beats/minute at 5–6 weeks of gestation to 140 beats/minute at 8–9 weeks of gestation. Embryonic heart rate has a high sensitivity for the prediction of miscarriage when the heart rate is less than the fifth percentile for gestational age. A heart rate below 85 beats/minute has been described as an indicator of impending embryonic loss.[32] However, it is important to be cautious when diagnosing miscarriage based on a bradycardic embryo, since a very small embryo (CRL 2–5 mm) can start off with a heart rate less than 100 beats/minute (Figure 3.12).

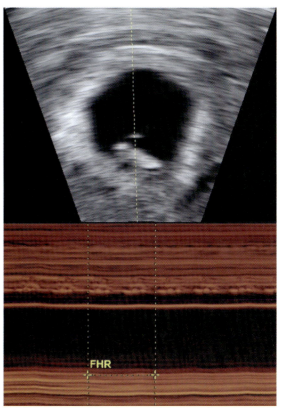

FIGURE 3.12 **Embryonic heart rate measurement using M-mode**

Role of biochemical markers

Biochemical markers are not used routinely in the diagnosis of miscarriage. However, they have played a role in predicting viability, particularly in identifying early pregnancy failure in pregnancies of unknown location. Serum human chorionic gonadotrophin (hCG) and progesterone are the two most commonly used biochemical markers. Novel biochemical markers that may assist in improving prediction of pregnancy outcome, such as inhibin A, have also been identified in more recent studies.

Human chorionic gonadotrophin

hCG levels in maternal serum double every 1.4–1.6 days from the time of first detection to the 35th day of pregnancy and then every 2.0–2.7 days from the 35th day to the 42nd day of pregnancy.[33] It has been well documented that slower hCG doubling times are associated with miscarriage.[34] However, the absolute levels of serum hCG cannot be used to discriminate between viable and non-viable pregnancies.[35] The half-life of hCG is between 32 and 37 hours, and it is common to find high levels in women with a history of recent early pregnancy failure. Owing to the wide range of serum hCG levels in early pregnancy, it is not possible to specify an optimal level below which the diagnosis of miscarriage is certain.

Serial measurements of hCG have been used in the assessment of pregnant women with non-diagnostic scans ('pregnancies of unknown location'). These studies have shown that declining hCG levels can diagnose a compete miscarriage with a sensitivity of between 93% and 97%.[36,37]

Progesterone

Serum progesterone in early pregnancy is mainly produced by the corpus luteum. Secretion of progesterone is controlled by hCG, which is produced by trophoblasts. Progesterone has a very short half-life and any abnormalities in trophoblast secretion of hCG have a rapid effect on serum progesterone levels. Therefore, serum progesterone levels can be used as a reliable indicator of trophoblastic function. For example, in women with ultrasound diagnosis of an empty gestational sac, the probability of pregnancy viability can be estimated using a logistic regression model that takes into account maternal age, size of the gestational sac and serum progesterone levels.[10] Progesterone is seen as the most powerful predictor of pregnancy outcome in this model, with a level under 25 nmol/l indicating embryonic demise. However, occasional cases of normal pregnancy have been reported in women with very low serum progesterone levels. Therefore, measurement of serum progesterone can be used to assess the risk of miscarriage, but it should not be used on its own as the definite diagnostic test to diagnose miscarriage.

Inhibin A

Inhibin A has an even shorter half-life (45 minutes) than hCG or progesterone, which should make it more sensitive in recognising trophoblastic failure. Studies have demonstrated decreased levels of inhibin A in missed miscarriages and complete miscarriages compared with controls.[38,39] However, in practice, inhibin A used in conjunction with hCG and progesterone does not show increased sensitivity compared with using hCG and progesterone only.[40] Further studies are needed focusing on the role of inhibin A in early pregnancy prior to its use as a diagnostic tool.

Conclusion

Transvaginal ultrasonography has revolutionised the diagnosis and management of early pregnancy complications. In normal pregnancies, a single ultrasound scan can reassure women that their risk of suffering early pregnancy failure is very low. Most cases of miscarriage can be diagnosed on a single examination, which helps with counselling and facilitates appropriate treatment. However, it is important to be aware that diagnostic errors may occur, which in the most severe cases could result in unintentional terminations of wanted pregnancies. It is vital that early pregnancy units have strict rules in place to avoid diagnostic errors occurring; in addition, access to experienced senior clinicians should be available in cases where the diagnosis is unclear. When ultrasound findings are not conclusive, the use of biochemical markers can play an important role. However, interpretation of the results of blood tests is not always easy and each unit should put in place clear protocols for the diagnosis and management of suspected early pregnancy failure based on the results of biochemical measurements.

References

1 Hemminki E. Treatment of miscarriage: current practice and rationale. *Obstet Gynecol* 1998;91:247–53.

2 Royal College of Obstetricians and Gynaecologists. *Management of early pregnancy loss.* Green-top Guideline No. 25. London: RCOG; 2006 [www.rcog.org.uk/womens-health/clinical-guidance/management-early-pregnancy-loss-green-top-25].

3 Shillito J, Walker J J. Early pregnancy assessment units. *Br J Hosp Med* 1997;58:505–9.

4 Bigrigg M A, Read M D. Management of women referred to early pregnancy assessment unit: care and cost effectiveness. *BMJ* 1991;302:577–9.

5 Farquharson R G, Jauniaux E, Exalto N; ESHRE Special Interest Group for Early Pregnancy (SIGEP). Updated and revised nomenclature for description of early pregnancy events. *Hum Reprod* 2005;20:3008–11.

6 Wieringa-de Waard M, Bonsel G J, Ankum W M, Vos J, Bindels PJ. Threatened miscarriage in general practice: diagnostic value of history taking and physical examination. *Br J Gen Pract* 2002;52:825–9.

7 Falco P, Zagonari S, Gabrielli S, Bevini M, Pilu G, Bovicelli L. Sonography of pregnancies with first-trimester bleeding and a small intrauterine gestational sac without a demonstrable embryo. *Ultrasound Obstet Gynecol* 2003;21:62–5.

8 Tongsong T, Wanapirak C, Srisomboon J, Sirichotiyakul S, Polsrisuthikul T, Pongsatha S. Transvaginal ultrasound in threatened abortions with empty gestational sacs. *Int J Gynaecol Obstet* 1994;46:297–301.

9 Nyberg D A, Laing F C, Filly R A. Threatened abortion: sonographic distinction of normal and abnormal gestation sacs. *Radiology* 1986;158:397–400.

10 Elson J, Salim R, Tailor A, Banerjee S, Zosmer N, Jurkovic D. Prediction of early pregnancy viability in the absence of an ultrasonically detectable embryo. *Ultrasound Obstet Gynaecol* 2003;21:57–61.

11 Levi C S, Lyons E A, Zheng X H, Lindsay D J, Holt S C. Endovaginal US: demonstration of cardiac activity in embryos of less than 5.0 mm in crown–rump length. *Radiology* 1990;176:71–4.

12 Ferrazzi E, Garbo S, Sulpizio P, Ghisoni L, Levi Setti P, Buscaglia M. Miscarriage diagnosis and gestational age estimation in the early first trimester of pregnancy: transabdominal versus transvaginal sonography. *Ultrasound Obstet Gynecol* 1993;3:36–41.

13 Hately W, Case J, Campbell S. Establishing the death of an embryo by ultrasound: report of a public inquiry with recommendations. *Ultrasound Obstet Gynecol* 1995;5:353–7.

14 Royal College of Radiologists, Royal College of Obstetricians and Gynaecologists. *Guidance on ultrasound procedures in early pregnancy*. London: RCR/RCOG; 1995.

15 Luise C, Jermy K, Collons W P, Bourne T H. Expectant management of incomplete, spontaneous first-trimester miscarriage: outcome according to initial ultraound criteria and value of follow-up visits. *Ultrasound Obstet Gynecol* 2002;19:580–2.

16 Jurkovic D. Three-dimensional ultrasound in gynecology: a critical evaluation. *Ultrasound Obstet Gynecol* 2002;19: 109–17.

17 Sairam S, Khare M, Michailidis G, Thilaganathan B. The role of ultrasound in the expectant management of early pregnancy loss. *Ultrasound Obstet Gynecol* 2001;17:506–9.

18 Nielsen S, Hahlin M. Expectant management of first-trimester spontaneous abortion. *Lancet* 1995;345:84–6.

19 Kurtz A B, Shlansky-Goldberg R D, Choi H Y, Needleman L, Wapner RJ, Goldberg BB. Detection of retained products of conception following spontaneous abortion in the first trimester. *J Ultrasound Med* 1991;10:387–95.

20 Rulin M C, Bornstein S G, Campbell J D. The reliability of ultrasonography in the management of spontaneous abortion, clinically thought to be complete: a prospective study. *Am J Obstet Gynecol* 1993;168:12–5.

21 Sawyer E, Ofuasia E, Ofili-Yebovi D, Helmy S, Gonzalez J, Jurkovic D. The value of measuring endometrial thickness and volume on transvaginal ultrasound scan for the diagnosis of incomplete miscarriage. *Ultrasound Obstet Gynecol* 2007;23:205–9.

22 Nybo Andersen A M, Wohlfahrt J, Christens P, Olsen J, Melbye M. Maternal age and fetal loss: population based register linkage study. *BMJ* 2000;320:1708–12.

23 Acharya G, Morgan H. First trimester, three-dimensional transvaginal ultrasound volumetry in normal pregnancies and spontaneous miscarriages. *Ultrasound Obstet Gynecol* 2002;19:575–9.

24 Levi C S, Lyons E A, Lindsay D J. Early diagnosis of nonviable pregnancy with endovaginal US. *Radiology* 1988;167:383–5.

25 Blaas H G, Eik-Nes S H, Bremnes J B. The growth of the human embryo. A longitudinal biometric assessment from 7 to 12 weeks of gestation. *Ultrasound Obstet Gynecol* 1998;12:346–54.

26 Lindsay D J, Lovett I S, Lyons E A, Levi C S, Zheng X H, Holt S C, et al. Yolk sac diameter and shape at endovaginal US: predictors of pregnancy outcome in the first trimester. *Radiology* 1992;183:115–8.

27 Makrydimas G, Sebire N J, Lolis D, Vlassis N, Nicolaides K H. Fetal loss following ultrasound diagnosis of a live fetus at 6–10 weeks of gestation. *Ultrasound Obstet Gynecol* 2003;22:368–72.

28 Grisolia G, Milano K, Pilu G, Banzi C, David C, Gabrielli S, et al. Biometry of early pregnancy with transvaginal sonography. *Ultrasound Obstet Gynecol* 1993;3:403–11.

29 McKenna K M, Feldstein V A, Goldstein R B , Filly R A. The empty amnion: a sign of early pregnancy failure. *J Ultrasound Med* 1995;14:117–21.

30 Reljic M. The significance of crown–rump length measurement for predicting adverse pregnancy outcome of threatened abortion. *Ultrasound Obstet Gynecol* 2001;17:510–2.

31 Mukri F, Bourne T, Bottomley C, Schoeb C, Kirk E, Papageorghiou A T. Evidence of early first-trimester growth restriction in pregnancies that subsequently end in miscarriage. *BJOG* 2008;115:1273–8.

32 Laboda L A, Estroff J A, Benacerraf B R. First trimester bradycardia. A sign of impending fetal loss. *J Ultrasound Med* 1989;8:561–3.

33 Pittaway D E, Reish R L, Wentz A C. Doubling times of human chorionic gonadotropin increase in early viable intrauterine pregnancies. *Am J Obstet Gynecol* 1985;152: 299–302

34 Lower A M, Yovich J L. The value of serum levels of oestradiol, progesterone and beta-human chorionic gonadotrophin in the prediction of early pregnancy loss. *Hum Reprod* 1992;7:711–7

35 Elson J, Tailor A, Salim R, Hillaby K, Dew T, Jurkovic D. Expectant management of miscarriage—prediction of outcome using ultrasound and novel biochemical markers. *Hum Reprod* 2005;20:2330 3.

36 Hahlin M, Thorburn J, Bryman I. The expectant management of early pregnancies of uncertain site. *Hum Reprod* 1995;10:1223–7.

37 Condous G, Kirk E, Van Calster B, Van Huffel S, Timmerman D, Bourne T. Failing pregnancies of unknown location: a prospective evaluation of the human chorionic gonadotrophin ratio. *BJOG* 2006;113:521–7.

38 Muttukrishna S. Role of inhibin in normal and high-risk pregnancy. *Semin Reprod Med* 2004;22:227–34.

39 Luisi S, Florio P, D'Antona, Severi F M, Sanseverino F, Danero S, et al. Maternal serum inhibin A levels are a marker of a viable trophoblast in incomplete and complete miscarriage. *Eur J Endocrinol* 2003;148:233–6.

40 Phipps M G, Hogan J W, Peipert J F, Lambert-Messerlian G M, Canick J A, Seifer DB. Progesterone, inhibin, and hCG multiple marker strategy to differentiate viable from nonviable pregnancies. *Obstet Gynecol* 2000;95:227–31.

4 Conservative and surgical management of miscarriage

Michelle Swer, Willem M Ankum and Davor Jurkovic

Introduction

For the past 50 years, the mainstay of treatment for the management of miscarriage has been surgical management, or the evacuation of retained products of conception. Until recently, up to 88% of women diagnosed with a miscarriage would be offered an evacuation of retained products of conception under general anaesthesia.[1] The rationale for surgical management was based on the assumption that the presence of a non-viable pregnancy within the uterus would increase the risk of infection and haemorrhage. In the past, these complications were more likely to develop from infected retained products of conception following poorly performed illegal abortions but, with the legalisation of abortion in developed countries, the introduction of antibiotics and a general improvement in women's health, these risks have decreased substantially. Over the past decade, there has been less emphasis on urgent surgical management and more on individualised treatment and patient choice between expectant, medical and semi-elective surgical treatment.

Expectant management

Expectant management is chosen by women because of a desire for a natural approach to management. It is becoming an increasingly popular option; in one observational study, 70% of women opted to wait for the pregnancy to resolve spontaneously.[2] The first randomised controlled trial of expectant management compared with surgical management of miscarriage, carried out by Nielsen and Hahlin, showed a 79% success rate for cases of incomplete or inevitable miscarriage when managed expectantly for 3 days, with no increased risk of pelvic infection or excessive bleeding.[3] Further studies have confirmed the safety and efficacy of expectant management.

Success rates

There are wide variations among studies regarding the success rate of expectant management. The rate of complete evacuation in individual trials ranges from 79% by 3 days[3] to 93% by 7 weeks.[2] The type of miscarriage is a significant factor in the effectiveness of this approach. A meta-analysis of data from randomised trials of expectant management showed higher success rates in incomplete miscarriages (80–94%), while miscarriages diagnosed as early embryonic demise had lower success rates (28–76%).[4] In the latter group, spontaneous miscarriage is often found to be more painful and less likely to be complete;[5] thus, expectant management may not necessarily be the most appropriate option in these cases.

The longer the follow-up, the greater the chance of success of completion, as seen in some studies.[6] However, for a reasonable chance of successful resolution (50%), 2 weeks is seen as an acceptable length of time to wait. The woman should be counselled to allow 2 weeks for expected completion, to avoid the risk of extra, unplanned visits. Nonetheless, should a woman wish to carry on with expectant management, there is no harm in continuing, provided there is no evidence of infection. It is important to give women clear, written information on what to expect and to ensure that continued support is available.

There is limited evidence on predicting the success of expectant management. A retrospective study in 1999 used five variables – progesterone, relative daily human chorionic gonadotrophin change, intrauterine diameter, serum CA125 and alphafetoprotein – in a logistic model to calculate the probability of successful outcome.[7] A 2008 study looked at the use of novel biochemical markers such as inhibin A and IGFBP-1, which have also been shown to be of value.[8] However, these parameters require the use of a computer program and all variables need to be entered, which is not feasible in a busy early pregnancy unit setting. The use of ultrasonographic features such as colour Doppler to assess the presence of intervillous blood flow has been shown to be helpful in the selection of patients.[9] The presence of the gestational sac or volume of retained products as measured on three-dimensional ultrasound do not appear to influence the chances of a successful outcome.[2,10]

Complications

The main disadvantage of expectant management is the unpredictability of the timescale and the final outcome. The risk of morbidity with unplanned surgical intervention is also higher compared with an elective procedure. One systematic review found no significant difference in the rate of complete evacuation between expectant management and surgery.[11] However, another systematic review of five trials concluded that women opting for expectant management were more likely to have incomplete emptying (RR 5.37, 95% CI 2.57–11.22) and were more at risk of additional or unplanned surgery (RR 4.78, 95% CI 1.99–11.48) than women electing for surgical management: the percentage of women needing unplanned surgery ranged from 2% to 20% in the expectant management group compared with 0% to 5% in the surgical group.[12]

The risk of excessive bleeding with expectant management is around 3%, which is similar to that reported with surgical management.[4] The duration of vaginal bleeding is also similar between the two groups, with a mean of 9.9 days with expectant management compared with 7.5 days with surgical management.[4]

The risk of infection is low with expectant management. The MIST trial, which compared expectant, medical and surgical management, showed no significant difference in the actual rate of infection among the three groups.[13]

Summary

Overall, expectant management is a safe and effective way to manage a miscarriage. It avoids the risks of surgery and general anaesthesia and gives the woman a sense of control over the situation. Studies have shown high patient satisfaction scores, with 71% of women happy to choose this management again should the situation arise.[14] The success rate in women diagnosed with early embryonic demise is not as high as that seen in women with incomplete miscarriage. In cases where the woman is asymptomatic an alternative option may be more suitable, unless the woman is determined to persevere with expectant management. The unpredictability of the outcome is the main disadvantage but with appropriate counselling and continued support it is a suitable and acceptable management option.

Medical management

Medical management for miscarriage has developed following the successful use of drugs as an alternative to surgical termination of pregnancy. Up to 20% of women opt for this approach.[15] A number of different regimens have been described and have been carried out by early pregnancy units in both inpatient and outpatient settings.

Treatment regimens

The most commonly used drug is the prostaglandin analogue misoprostol, which can be administered in either a single dose or divided doses. It is licensed for oral use only, but can be administered vaginally, sublingually or rectally. The vaginal route has a greater bioavailability[16] and has been shown to be more effective than the oral route,[17] although some studies have shown no significant difference in efficacy between the two routes.[18,19]

Mifepristone, an oral antiprogesterone drug, is thought to potentiate the effects of prostaglandins. It is licensed for softening and dilatation of the cervix prior to surgical termination and has been shown to increase the efficacy of misoprostol in therapeutic abortions.[20] It is sometimes used prior to the administration of misoprostol for miscarriage. However, the addition of mifepristone in medical management of miscarriage has not been shown to increase the success rate of misoprostol alone.[21,22]

Success rates

The success of medical management depends on the type of miscarriage, the drug dosage, the route of administration and the time allowed for products to be passed.

In initial observational studies, success rates were high for both early embryonic demise (93%) and incomplete miscarriage (94%).[15,23] However, further studies have shown success rates ranging from 70% to 96% for incomplete miscarriages and lower rates of 52–92% for embryonic demise.[16–21] For those diagnosed with embryonic demise, the success rates are higher for women who choose medical management than for those who opt for expectant management alone. However, for incomplete miscarriages there are similar outcomes for the two approaches.[13] In fact, medical intervention in this group is thought unlikely to improve the outcome.[5]

Vaginal misoprostol has been administered at doses of 400 micrograms, 600 micrograms and 800 micrograms in various trials. Route of administration and dosage were associated with differences in the success rates. Oral doses of 400 micrograms misoprostol given at 4-hourly intervals were found to be less effective than a single vaginal dose of 800 micrograms, with success rates of 50%[24] and 82%,[22] respectively. Higher doses have been advised for women diagnosed with early embryonic demise and in these cases concurrent use of mifepristone is thought to be useful.

However, success rates are also dependent on the duration of follow-up and the time allowed before surgical intervention is offered. One study showed that allowing a longer time for completion of miscarriage (10 days as opposed to 48 hours) with small repeated doses of misoprostol (200 micrograms four times daily for 5 days) administered on an outpatient basis resulted in similar rates to those obtained surgically (93% versus 100%).[25] However, this requires appropriate management in an outpatient setting as well as patient compliance.

Complications

The main adverse effects of prostaglandin use are gastrointestinal symptoms, including diarrhoea and vomiting, and increased bleeding. A meta-analysis of various dosages and routes of administration of misoprostol found a nausea rate of 23% and a diarrhoea rate of 18%.[11] Similar figures have been found in the published trials, despite the different dosages given, although there was less vomiting with the oral regimen but a comparable incidence of diarrhoea.[26] Nonetheless, the gastrointestinal symptoms are not severe enough to dissuade women from accepting medical management.[24]

The risk of heavy bleeding requiring emergency evacuation after treatment with misoprostol has been reported at 5%, with a higher risk in women who were also treated with mifepristone (11%).[27] The risk of blood transfusion in women pretreated with mifrepristone is 1%.[28] The infection rate with expectant management is 2% at 14 days and 3% at 8 weeks, which is similar to the figures reported for surgical management.[13]

In cases where medical management fails and surgery is carried out, there appear to be fewer surgery-related complications. This is thought to be because of the softening effect of the drugs on the cervix, which allows easier instrumentation of the uterus.[4]

Summary

Medical management of miscarriage, like expectant management, avoids the risks associated with surgery. Studies have shown that it offers faster completion of the miscarriage with higher success rates in those diagnosed with early embryonic demise. However, the failure rate is significant and there is also a risk of emergency surgery.

Medical management can be offered in the outpatient setting of early pregnancy units since it does not require women to be admitted. The treatment should be conducted preferably in designated rooms to allow some degree of privacy. However, medical management does require providing the woman with sufficient information and appropriate support when needed.

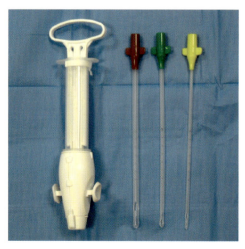

FIGURE 4.1 **A set for manual suction aspiration of retained products of conception**

Surgical management

Surgery remains the treatment of choice in women who present with excessive bleeding, are haemodynamically unstable, have signs of infected retained products of conception or have a provisional diagnosis of gestational trophoblastic disease. It is otherwise offered as an elective procedure for women who express an interest in surgical intervention since it is quick and may help with the woman's grieving process.

Surgical techniques

Curettage under general anaesthesia
Traditionally, metal curettage was the surgical technique used in the removal of retained products of conception under general anaesthesia. This method is still popular in developing countries but is not used in routine clinical practice in the UK, where suction curettage (or vacuum aspiration) is now the method of choice. A Cochrane review comparing suction curettage with sharp curettage in incomplete miscarriages showed significantly reduced intraoperative blood loss, shorter operating time and less postoperative pain in women who were operated on using suction curettage in comparison with metal curettage.[29]

Manual vacuum aspiration under local anaesthesia
The use of manual vacuum aspiration was first described in the 1970s for surgical treatment of presumed incomplete miscarriages. It is more widely used in the USA and developing countries than in the UK, where this technique is mainly used for early first-trimester terminations. Manual vacuum aspiration has been carried out using systemic analgesia (intravenous alfentanil and midazolam) or patient-controlled analgesia (alfentanil and propofol) in operating theatres.[30] This procedure can also be performed in an outpatient setting under local anaesthesia, avoiding the need for an operating theatre.[31] The benefits of outpatient procedures are increased safety owing

to decreased surgical and anaesthesia risks, minimal social interruption and reduced costs.

There is no consensus in the literature regarding selection criteria and suitability of women for evacuation of retained products of conception under local anaesthesia. The selection criteria listed in Box 4.1 are used by the authors.

Cervical priming is used to minimise pain and increase the chances of success. Sublingual misoprostol has been used in one study, showing 94.7% efficacy.[31] Dilapan-S™ (FEMA International), a 3 mm hygroscopic cervical dilator, can also be used. This is inserted at least 4 hours before the procedure and removed at the time of evacuation. A study comparing the efficacy and acceptability of three principles of cervical priming on women undergoing first-trimester terminations showed the use of misoprostol gel and Dilapan-S to be equally effective, with the Dilapan-S causing more discomfort at the time of insertion but fewer adverse effects of uterine contractions.[32]

Manual vacuum aspiration is carried out in a dedicated treatment room by a doctor with the assistance of a nurse. A paracervical block is administered with 1% lignocaine. A Karman suction curette is used and negative pressure obtained using a modified 50 ml locking syringe (Figure 4.1). This is carried out under transabdominal ultrasound guidance to ensure that the procedure is completed (Figures 4.2 and 4.3).

Manual vacuum aspiration under local anaesthesia is an effective surgical alternative that can be offered to women who want early resolution of their miscarriage but wish to avoid general anaesthesia. It also has advantages for the healthcare provider by reducing hospital costs, waiting times and hospital stays.

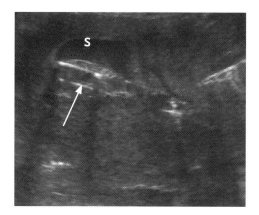

FIGURE 4.2 **Suction aspiration under ultrasound guidance**

The aspiration cannula appears hyperechoic and is easily identifiable within the uterine cavity (arrow) below the gestational sac (S).

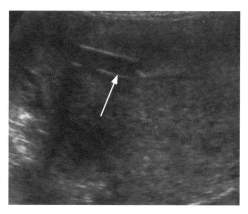

FIGURE 4.3 **The uterine cavity is empty at the end of the procedure, with the arrow pointing to the cannula**

Success rates

Surgical management of miscarriage is the most efficacious option in the management of miscarriage. In a meta-analysis of women undergoing surgical curettage as the control group in randomised controlled trials of expectant and medical management, the rate of complete evacuation was 97%.[11] There is a low risk of the woman needing further intervention or requiring unplanned hospital admission. The type of miscarriage does not dictate success rates; surgical technique does not appear to affect success rates either.

Complications

The main risks of surgical management are retained products of conception, infection and bleeding. Other less common risks to be aware of are perforation to the uterus, cervical damage, intrauterine adhesions and intra-abdominal trauma. Women should also be informed about the risk of vasovagal reaction and pain and the possibility of transfer to an operating theatre when the procedure is performed in the clinic under local anaesthesia.

The risk of retained products of conception is lower in surgical patients than in women undergoing medical management or expectant management, with rates of 1–3% for surgical patients.[33] The intraoperative use of ultrasonography has been suggested since the 1980s, especially in cases where there is acute anteflexion or retroflexion or cervical stenosis.[34] More recent studies have shown that the number of incomplete evacuations is significantly lower in women who have the procedure performed with the aid of ultrasound.[33] The routine use of intraoperative ultrasound can therefore help to ensure the completeness of uterine evacuation and to reduce the overall complication rate.

The infection rates reported in randomised controlled trials comparing medical and surgical management are about 4–5%,[27] although larger trials suggest rates of 3–4%.[4] The MIST trial (miscarriage treatment trial) looked at the incidence of infection in women managed surgically, expectantly and medically; the results showed no difference in the rate of infections among the three groups.[13] There is insufficient evidence to recommend antibiotic prophylaxis prior to surgery, and the RCOG Green-top Guidelines on the management of early pregnancy loss recommend prophylaxis on an individual basis.[35] However, it is recommended that all at-risk women be screened for *Chlamydia trachomatis*.

Excessive bleeding requiring blood transfusion is less likely to occur with surgical management than with medical or expectant management.[11] It is more likely to be anticipated in cases of undiagnosed gestational trophoblastic disease or cervical pregnancies. This can be prevented by adequate preoperative preparation including cross-matching blood units and easy access to uterotonics such as misoprostol and syntocinon infusion. Fetomaternal haemorrhage can occur in surgical procedures and it is therefore recommended to give anti-D to all non-sensitised RH-negative women who undergo evacuation.

Cervical damage and uterine perforation are uncommon complications, with rates of 0.3% and 1.9% quoted, respectively.[24] Cervical damage can arise from dilatation of the cervix or use of instruments to stabilise the cervix for instrumentation. Uterine perforation should be suspected in women who present with symptoms of shock postoperatively or who develop an acute abdomen or irregular bleeding. Ultrasound findings in these cases show blood in the uterine cavity and/or evidence of retained products of conception. The use of cervical priming is seen as a means of reducing the risk of uterine perforation.

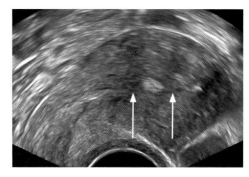

FIGURE 4.4 **A case of intrauterine adhesions: a longitudinal section of the uterus showing an interrupted endometrial echo (arrows), which is typical of adhesions**

Intrauterine adhesions can occur as a result of trauma to the endometrium during surgical curettage and can form in up to 8% of women.[36] Ultrasound features show a dense area of adhesions in the uterine cavity (Figure 4.4). Adhesions can be a cause of recurrent miscarriage in women who have had previous uterine surgery and should be suspected in women who present with symptoms of menstrual irregularity.

Summary

Surgical management is the most successful option for the management of miscarriage. Although conservative management has gained in popularity in recent years, 30% of women opt for surgery as their preferred primary treatment option.[2] In addition, 30–40% of women required surgical evacuation because of unsuccessful conservative management. The introduction of evacuation under local anaesthesia may further enhance the role of surgery in the management of miscarriage, as many women try to avoid surgery because of a fear of general anaesthesia.

Conclusion

The management of miscarriage has changed over the past 10 years, with an increase in the number of management options offered when a patient is haemodynamically stable. Each has its own advantages and disadvantages. There is no concern regarding the risk of infection and impact on subsequent fertility. The importance lies in ensuring that the woman is provided with comprehensive information on each type of management, careful counselling and access to emergency medical support so that she is able to choose the option that best suits her specific requirements and expectations.

References

1 Hemminki E. Treatment of miscarriage: current practice and rationale. *Obstet Gynecol* 1998;91:247–53.

2 Luise C, Jermy K, May C, Costello G, Collins W P, Bourne TH. Outcome of expectant management of spontaneous first trimester miscarriage: observational study. *BMJ* 2002;324:873–5.

3 Nielsen S, Hahlin M. Expectant management of first-trimester spontaneous abortion. *Lancet* 1995;345:84–6.

4 Graziosi G C, Mol B W, Ankum W M, Bruinse H W. Management of early pregnancy loss. *Int J Gynecol Obstet* 2004;86:337–46.

5 Condous G. The management of early pregnancy complications. *Best Pract Res Clin Obstet Gynaecol* 2004;18:37–57.

6 Sairam S, Khare M, Michailidis G, Thilaganathan B. The role of ultrasound in the expectant management of early pregnancy loss. *Ultrasound Obstet Gynecol* 2001;17:506–9.

7 Nielsen S, Hahlin M, Odén A. Using a logistic model to identify women with first-trimester spontaneous abortion suitable for expectant management. *Br J Obstet Gynaecol* 1996;103:1230–5.

8 Elson J, Tailor A, Salim R, Hillaby K, Dew T, Jurkovic D. Expectant management of miscarriage–prediction of outcome using ultrasound and novel biochemical markers. *Hum Reprod* 2005;20:2330–3.

9 Schwärzler P, Holden D, Nielsen S, Hahlin M, Sladkevicius P, Bourne TH. The conservative management of first-trimester miscarriages and the use of colour Doppler sonography for patient selection. *Hum Reprod* 1999;14:1341–5.

10 Acharya G, Morgan H. First trimester, three-dimensional transvaginal ultrasound volumetry in normal pregnancies and spontaneous miscarriages. *Ultrasound Obstet Gynecol* 2002;19:575–9.

11 Sotiriadis A, Makrydimas G, Papatheodorou S, Ioannidis JP. Expectant, medical, or surgical management of first-trimester miscarriage: a meta-analysis. *Obstet Gynecol* 2005;105:1104–13.

12 Nanda K, Peloggia A, Grimes D, Lopez L, Nanda G. Expectant care versus surgical treatment for miscarriage. *Cochrane Database Syst Rev* 2006;(2):CD003518.

13 Trinder J, Brocklehurst P, Porter R, Read M, Vyas S, Smith L. Management of miscarriage: expectant, medical, or surgical? Results of randomised controlled trial (miscarriage treatment [MIST] trial). *BMJ* 2006;332:1235–40.

14 Wieringa-de Waard M, Bindels P J, Vos J, Bonsel G J, Stalmeier P F, Ankum W M. Patient preferences for expectant management vs. surgical evacuation in first-trimester uncomplicated miscarriage. *J Clin Epidemiol* 2004;57:167–73

15 el-Refaey H, Hinshaw K, Henshaw R, Smith N, Templeton A. Medical management of missed abortion and anembryonic pregnancy. *BMJ* 1992;305:1399.

16 Zieman M, Fong S K, Benowitz N L, Banskter D, Darney PD. Absorption kinetics of misoprostol with oral or vaginal administration. *Obstet Gynecol* 1997;90:88–92.

17 Crenin M D, Moyer R, Guido R. Misoprostol for medical evacuation of early pregnancy failure. *Obstet Gynecol* 1997;89:768–72.

18 Tang O S, Ho P C. The use of misoprostol for early pregnancy failure. *Curr Opin Obstet Gynecol* 2006;18:581–6.

19 Ngoc N T, Blum J, Westheimer E, Quan T T, Winikoff B. Medical treatment of missed abortion using misoprostol. *Int J Gynaecol Obstet* 2004;87:138–42.

20 Kulier R, Gülmezoglu A M, Hofmeyr G J, Cheng L N, Campana A. Medical methods for first trimester abortion. *Cochrane Database Syst Rev* 2004;(1):CD002855.

21 Nielsen S, Hahlin M, Platz-Christensen J. Randomised trial comparing expectant with medical management for first-trimester miscarriages. *Br J Obstet Gynaecol* 1999;106:804–7.

22 Demetroulis C, Saridogan E, Kunde D, Naftalin A A. A prospective randomized control trial comparing medical and surgical treatment for early pregnancy failure. *Hum Reprod* 2001;16:365–9.

23 Henshaw R C, Naji S A, Russell I T, Templeton A A. Comparison of medical abortion with surgical vacuum aspiration: women's preferences and acceptability of treatment. *BMJ* 1993;307:714–7

24 Chung T K, Lee D T, Cheung L P, Haines C J, Chang A M. Spontaneous abortion: a randomized, controlled trial comparing surgical evacuation with conservative management using misoprostol. *Fertil Steril* 1999;71:1054–9.

25 Sahin H G, Sahin H A, Kocer M. Randomized outpatient clinical trial of medical evacuation and surgical curettage in incomplete miscarriage. *Eur J Contracept Reprod Health Care* 2001;6:141–4.

26 Nielson J P, Hickey M, Vazquez J. Medical treatment for early fetal death (less than 24 weeks). *Cochrane Database Syst Rev* 2006;(3):CD002253.

27 Grønlund A, Grønlund L, Clevin L, Andersen B, Palmgren N, Lidegaard Ø. Management of missed abortion: comparison of medical treatment with either mifepristone + misoprostol or misoprostol alone with surgical evacuation. A multi-center trial in Copenhagen county, Denmark. *Acta Obstet Gynecol Scand* 2002;81:1060–5.

28 Blohm F, Fridén B, Platz-Christensen J J, Milsom I, Nielsen S. Expectant management of first-trimester miscarriage in clinical practice. *Acta Obstet Gynecol Scand* 2003;82:654–8.

29 Forna F, Gülmezoglu A M. Surgical procedures to evacuate incomplete abortion. *Cochrane Database Syst Rev* 2001;(1):CD001993.

30 Gazvani R, Honey E, MacLennan F M, Templeton A. Manual vacuum aspiration (MVA) in the management of first trimester pregnancy loss. *Eur J Obstet Gynecol Reprod Biol* 2004;112:197–200.

31 Milingos D S, Mathur M, Smith N C, Ashok P W. Manual vacuum aspiration: a safe alternative for the surgical management of early pregnancy loss. *BJOG* 2009;116:1268–71.

32 Chen F C, Bergann A, Krosse J, Merholz A, David M. Isosorbide mononitrate vaginal gel versus misoprostol vaginal gel versus Dilapan-S for cervical ripening before first trimester curettage. *Eur J Obstet Gynecol Reprod Biol* 2008;138:176–9.

33 Debby A, Malinger G, Harow E, Golan A, Glezerman M. Transvaginal ultrasound after first-trimester uterine evacuation reduces the incidence of retained products of conception. *Ultrasound Obstet Gynecol* 2006;27:61–4.

34 Goldenberg R L, Davis R O, Hill D. The use of real-time ultrasound as an aid during difficult therapeutic abortion procedures. *Am J Obstet Gynecol* 1984;148:826–7.

35 Royal College of Obstetricians and Gynaecologists. Green-top Guideline No. 25: *The management of early pregnancy loss*. London: RCOG; 2006 [www.rcog.org.uk/womens-health/clinical-guidance/management-early-pregnancy-loss-green-top-25].

36 Tam W H, Tsui M H, Lok I H, Yip S K, Yuen P M, Chung T K. Long-term reproductive outcome subsequent to medical versus surgical treatment for miscarriage. *Hum Reprod* 2005;20:3355–9.

5 Management of hyperemesis gravidarum

Sangeeta Suri

Introduction

Nausea and vomiting are common in pregnancy, affecting 70–80% of women in early pregnancy.[1] Up to one-third of all pregnant women have to take time off work on at least one occasion as a result of nausea and vomiting of pregnancy.[2] However, it is generally a mild condition and tends to resolve spontaneously.

By contrast, hyperemesis gravidarum (HG) is a severe intractable form of nausea and vomiting that occurs typically in the first trimester of pregnancy, leads to fluid and electrolyte imbalances, weight loss and ketonuria and is severe enough to require hospital admission.[3] It affects approximately 0.3–2.0% of pregnancies,[3–5] typically occurring between 4 and 10 weeks of gestation, with resolution of the symptoms by 20 weeks of gestation. However, in approximately 10% of affected women the symptoms persist throughout pregnancy.[1] Nowadays, HG rarely causes serious morbidity, but before the advent of intravenous fluids for treatment in the 1930s the mortality rate from this condition was 159 deaths per million births in the UK.[6]

Epidemiology

Epidemiological studies have identified that women with HG are more likely to be non-white race, younger and non-smokers with a previous or family history of the condition. They may have co-existing medical disorders and their pregnancies are more likely to be complicated by molar pregnancy, multiple gestation or Down syndrome (Table 5.1).[4,7]

Aetiology

The pathophysiology of HG is poorly understood. Various endocrine, mechanical, infective and psychological factors have been implicated, although no one theory has been shown to apply to all cases. The aetiology is therefore likely to involve complex interactions between a number of these factors.

TABLE 5.1 **Risk factors associated with hyperemesis gravidarum**

	Risk factors
Demographics	Non-white race
	Younger maternal age
	Non-smoker
	Nulliparous
Current pregnancy	Multiple pregnancy
	Molar pregnancy
	Down syndrome
	Female fetus
Other factors	Family history of hyperemesis gravidarum
	Previous hyperemesis gravidarum
	Asthma
	Hyperthyroidism
	Diabetes
	Psychological stress

Endocrine factors

Human chorionic gonadotrophin

Human chorionic gonadotrophin (hCG) is often assumed to be the most likely cause of HG. This is because there is a strong temporal association between the peak incidence of hyperemesis and peak serum hCG levels in early pregnancy. In addition, HG is more likely to occur in pregnancies with high hCG levels, such as multiple and molar pregnancies.[8,9]

A systematic review of 15 published prospective comparative studies on the possible causes of HG found that, in 11 of the 15 studies, recorded serum hCG levels were significantly higher in women with HG compared with the control groups.[10] It has been suggested that hCG causes hyperemesis through a stimulating effect on secretory processes in the upper gastrointestinal tract. An alternative suggestion is that, in view of its structural similarity to thyroid-stimulating hormone (TSH), it causes hyperemesis through its effect on the TSH receptor[11,12] (see below).

Other hormones, particularly estradiol and progesterone, have also been considered as causative factors in HG, but to date the evidence has not supported a causal relationship.[13]

Thyroid hormones

In early pregnancy the thyroid gland is physiologically stimulated and occasionally this leads to gestational transient thyrotoxicosis, a condition where a woman is clinically euthyroid but her serum thyroid hormone concentrations deviate from the normal range (high thyroxine, low TSH). This is thought to occur as a result of the structural similarity between hCG and TSH (common alpha subunit), which may lead to hCG-stimulating thyroid activity.[14] In 11 of 15 prospective reviews there were significantly higher thyroxine levels in the hyperemesis group compared with control groups, and nine of 13 studies demonstrated significantly higher TSH levels in the HG group.[10] In gestational transient thyrotoxicosis, the abnormal thyroid function tests return to normal by 18 weeks.[14]

Mechanical factors

An alternative theory as to the cause of HG is that it may result from distension of the upper gastrointestinal tract as a result of excessive secretion and accumulation of fluid in the gut lumen leading to vomiting. Additionally, sex steroids reduce small intestinal motility and gastric emptying times, which may cause nausea,[15,16] although as steroid levels increase as the pregnancy progresses it is not clear why vomiting is generally confined to the first trimester. However, one study evaluated the gastric emptying times of women with HG against controls and found an increase in gastric emptying in women with HG.[17]

Infective factors

An increased incidence of infection with *Helicobacter pylori* has been found in women with HG compared with asymptomatic controls, with the density of colonisation correlating to the severity of symptoms.[18] There have also been reports of resolution of HG symptoms after treatment for *H. pylori* in women who were resistant to standard treatment for HG.[18,19] *H. pylori* has therefore been proposed as an aetiological factor in HG. However, it has also been suggested that the infection may be a result of HG, owing to the damage caused to the gastric mucosa by persistent vomiting,[10] rather than an actual cause. Additionally, it should be remembered that the majority of pregnant women with *H. pylori* remain asymptomatic.

Psychological factors

In the past, persistent vomiting in pregnancy was thought to be an expression of resentment or ambivalence towards pregnancy. Factors associated with this included emotional immaturity and strong mother dependence.[20] Investigators have recently opposed this theory, stating that the psychological stress experienced by these women may be a result of HG rather than a cause.[21]

Diagnosis and investigations

The diagnosis of hyperemesis is one of exclusion. No single test exists that will confirm the condition. The diagnosis is usually made when the woman's history suggests intractable vomiting and inability to tolerate any food or fluids in the presence of ketonuria, which generally occurs during the first trimester. It is important to take a detailed history to exclude symptoms of other causes of vomiting, such as associated diarrhoea for a gastrointestinal tract infection, frequency and dysuria for a urinary tract infection or abdominal pain for pancreatitis or peptic ulcers. Enquiries should also be made about epigastric pain and haematemesis (secondary to Mallory–Weiss tears) as well as associated symptoms such as ptyalism (inability to swallow), spitting and weight loss.

The duration of vomiting is relevant, as persistent vomiting can result in thiamine deficiency and increase the risk of complications (specifically Wernicke encephalopathy).

Examination findings will often show evidence of weight loss and signs of dehydration with postural hypotension and tachycardia.[22] The evaluation should include a complete abdominal examination to assess for tenderness and palpable masses.

Investigations will usually reveal hyponatraemia, hypokalaemia, low serum urea and metabolic hypochloraemic alkalosis as a result of excessive vomiting. A significant proportion of women will have moderately elevated transaminases, which tend to return to normal as the hyperemesis is treated. A proportion of affected women will have thyroid function abnormalities; however, the majority of these women will be clinically euthyroid, with levels returning to normal without treatment by approximately 18 weeks of gestation.[14] Additional investigations will show a raised haematocrit and possibly anaemia due to vitamin B_6 and B_{12} deficiency.

There should be evidence of ketonuria to confirm the diagnosis, and the urine is routinely screened to exclude infection.

An ultrasound scan should be performed to confirm the gestation and exclude risk factors associated with hyperemesis, such as multiple or molar pregnancies (Figures 5.1 and 5.2).

Complications

Maternal complications

There were three maternal deaths due to HG recorded in the Confidential Enquiry into Maternal Deaths in the UK between 1991 and 1993.[23] Two of those deaths were probably the result of Wernicke encephalopathy and one was the result of aspiration of vomit. No deaths have been reported since.

Nowadays the main concern with hyperemesis is malnutrition and the complications that occur as a result.

Vitamin B_6 and B_{12} deficiency

Vitamin B_6 (pyridoxine) and B_{12} (cyanocobalamin) deficiency can occur with HG and result in anaemia or peripheral neuropathy; however, there is little evidence to recommend routine administration of these vitamins to prevent complications of this disease.

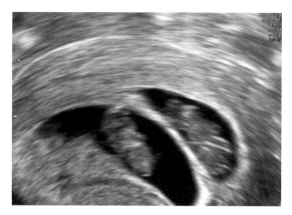

FIGURE 5.1 **Ultrasound scan of a dichorionic diamniotic twin pregnancy in a woman presenting with hyperemesis at 7 weeks of gestation**

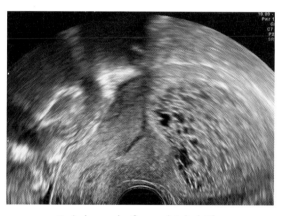

FIGURE 5.2 **Typical example of a complete hydatiform mole in a woman with history of hyperemesis and 10 weeks of amenorrhoea**

Wernicke's encephalopathy

Wernicke's encephalopathy is a rare, potentially fatal complication of HG that occurs as a result of vitamin B_1 (thiamine) deficiency. It can be precipitated by carbohydrate-rich foods or dextrose infusions.

The typical presentation – a triad of ocular signs, ataxia and a confusional state – is seen in approximately 47% of cases.[24] However, the presentation is not always typical and some signs may be absent. The condition tends to present at a mean gestational age of 14 weeks, with vomiting and feeding difficulties occurring approximately 7 weeks before the onset of symptoms.[24]

The condition is often underdiagnosed, but it should be suspected in women who present with a prolonged history of hyperemesis and neurological symptoms. Findings include abnormal liver function and reduced erythrocyte transketolase (a thiamine-dependent enzyme) activity, although this is of limited practical value as a test because the measurement is rarely available. Magnetic resonance imaging is the gold standard for diagnosis and shows symmetrical lesions around the aqueduct cerebri and fourth ventricle.[25] Treatment should not be delayed pending investigations but rather should be commenced on the basis of the clinical signs. Thiamine should be given parenterally if there is any doubt about the diagnosis; the drug is generally harmless, while the condition is not. Symptom resolution does not occur quickly. It may require months of therapy and in 60% of cases there will be some residual impairment.[24] The fetal loss rate including terminations is nearly 50%.

Hyponatraemia

Hyponatraemia is very common in HG. Symptoms rarely occur until the serum sodium is less than 120 mmol/l and are more usually associated with values around 110 mmmol/l. The signs and symptoms are non-specific and include anorexia, headache, confusion and restlessness leading to drowsiness, myoclonic jerks, generalised convulsions and, eventually, coma.

Rapid correction of serum sodium is dangerous and can result in osmotic demyelination syndrome (central pontine myelinolysis), which is characterised by loss of myelin in the pontine neurones. The classic symptoms are confusion, dysarthria and dysphagia, spastic quadriparesis and paralysis, which can reflect damage to the corticospinal and corticobulbar tracts.[26]

Mallory–Weiss tears

The prolonged vomiting in hyperemesis may result in linear mucosal tears at the oesophagogastric junction (Mallory–Weiss tears) and haematemesis. In the majority of cases these will resolve; however, if they persist or result in anaemia, further gastrointestinal investigations should be performed.

Venous thromboembolism

Pregnancy, immobility and dehydration are all significant risk factors for the development of thrombosis in women with HG. While there is little guidance with regard to thromboprophylaxis in women who develop hyperemesis, it seems reasonable to encourage the use of thromboembolic stockings and consider the use of low-molecular-weight heparin on an individual basis.

Termination of pregnancy

Surveys have shown that there is an increased likelihood that women suffering with hyperemesis will consider a termination of pregnancy.[27]

Depression

HG is strongly associated with depression. Observational studies have shown that up to 50% of women with nausea and vomiting in early pregnancy are found to have potential psychiatric problems.[28] Whether earlier psychological input would have an impact on the condition is not known.

Fetal complications

While it was initially thought that hyperemesis was not associated with any adverse fetal outcomes, several studies have shown that babies born to women with HG have an increased rate of prematurity, being small for gestational age and American Pediatric Gross Assessment Record scores less than 7 at 5 minutes.[4,29] The rate of these complications was higher in babies born to women with HG who had less than 7 kg weight gain throughout their pregnancy. Women with HG and weight gain greater than 7 kg had similar rates of preterm birth to women without HG.[29]

Hyperemesis also appears to exert a protective effect, with several studies reporting lower early pregnancy losses in women with HG compared with asymptomatic controls.[30,31]

Management

Severe nausea and vomiting are among the leading causes of hospitalisation in pregnancy. The aims of any treatment plan are to manage the symptoms of nausea and vomiting, correct dehydration and electrolyte abnormalities and prevent and/or treat the complications associated with this condition (Figure 5.3). Any woman who is ketotic and unable to maintain adequate hydration should be admitted to hospital, although several units have successfully introduced a policy of managing these women as day cases (Table 5.2).[32]

Dietary advice

There is a general tendency to advise women who are experiencing nausea and vomiting in pregnancy to eat small, more frequent dry meals; however, there is no evidence to support this advice.

TABLE 5.2 **Protocol for outpatient management of hyperemesis gravidarum**

Inclusion criteria:

- Severe dehydration
- Inability to retain fluids orally
- >2+ ketones on dipstick
- Electrolyte imbalance

Exclusion criteria:

- Maternal request
- Diabetes
- Abnormal thyroid function test, liver function test and urea and electrolytes

On admission:

- Clinical examination
- Weight
- Blood pressure
- Heart rate
- Temperature

Investigations:

- Full bood count
- Urea and electrolytes
- Liver function test
- Thyroid function test
- Random blood sugar
- Urine microscopy
- Pelvic scan

Intravenous rehydration: 2 litres of physiological (0.9%) saline with 20 mmol KCl/bag over 4–6 hours

Antiemetic therapy (intravenous or intramuscular)

Hourly observations

Dietary advice

Discharge home with antiemetics, folic acid and oral thiamine

Contact point if symptoms return

Reassurance

Intravenous fluid replacement

Treating dehydration and electrolyte replacement are crucial to the management of hyperemesis. Dextrose-containing solutions should be avoided as they increase the chance of precipitating Wernicke's encephalopathy by increasing the body's requirement for thiamine and because the amount of sodium contained in dextrose-containing solutions is not sufficient to correct the hyponatraemia (Table 5.3).

Potassium chloride can be added to saline if necessary, depending on the patient's serum sodium and potassium levels. There is no place for the use of sodium chloride in higher concentrations than standard (1.8%), even in cases of severe hyponatraemia, as this may result in too rapid a correction of the sodium levels with the risk of central pontine myelinosis. The rise in serum sodium concentration should not exceed 10 mmol/l in 24 hours.

Fluid and electrolyte regimens should be adapted daily and titrated against daily electrolyte and fluid balance measurements. Women should also be weighed at regular intervals.

Thiamine (vitamin B$_1$) supplementation

Thiamine supplementation should be given to any woman suffering with prolonged vomiting. The requirement for thiamine increases during pregnancy to 1.5 mg daily.[33] It should be remembered that, generally, by the time these women present, they have been vomiting for 1–2 weeks. If they can tolerate tablets, thiamine can be given as thiamine hydrochloride tablets 25–50 mg three times a day. Alternatively, if oral intake cannot be tolerated, thiamine can be given intravenously as part of a multivitamin infusion on a weekly basis, such as Pabrinex® (Archimedes, Reading, UK), which contains 250 mg of thiamine hydrochloride and 50 mg of pyridoxine hydrochloride per pair of ampoules.

Treatment of Wernicke's encephalopathy requires much higher doses of thiamine.

FIGURE 5.3 **Management plan for hyperemesis gravidarum**

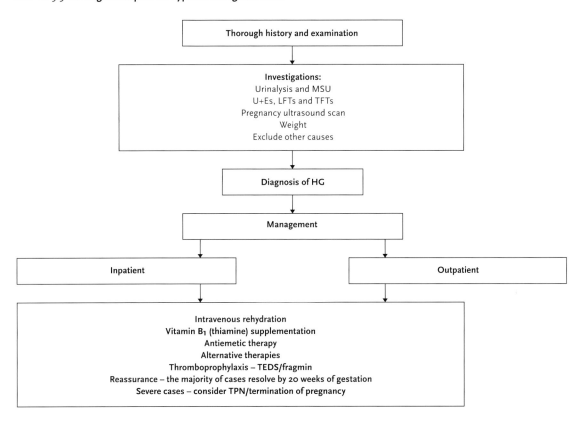

HG = hyperemesis gravidarum | LFTs = liver function tests | MSU = mid-stream urine |
TEDS = thromboembolism-deterrent stockings | TFTs = thyroid function tests | TPN = total parenteral nutrition |
U+Es = urea and electrolytes.

Antiemetic therapy

In the majority of cases women will respond to fluid replacement and vitamin supplementation; however, if this fails, consideration should be given
to antiemetic therapy. Understandably, in the post-thalidomide era there has

TABLE 5.3 **Sodium content of intravenous fluid replacement**

Intravenous fluid	Sodium content (mmol / l)
5% dextrose	0
Dextrose saline	30
Hartmann's solution (sodium chloride 0.6%)	131
Physiological saline (sodium chloride 0.9%)	150

been anxiety and reluctance to prescribe antiemetics, but extensive data exist showing no evidence of teratogenicity of the drugs studied.[34,35]

Antihistamine antiemetics

Antihistamines are effective against nausea and vomiting for many conditions. The two types commonly used in the UK are promethazine (10–20 mg orally three times a day; 25–50 mg intramuscularly, maximum 100 mg/day) and cyclizine (50 mg intravenously three times a day). The older antihistamines have a sedating effect; cyclizine perhaps less so than promethazine. This group is generally used in first-line treatment.

Phenothiazines

Phenothiazines are dopamine antagonists that act centrally by inhibiting the chemoreceptor trigger zone as well as having an action on the dopamine receptors in the gastrointestinal tract. Prochlorperazine (5–10 mg orally three times a day; 12.5 mg intramuscularly three times a day) is less sedating than chlorpromazine. Severe dystonic reactions occasionally occur with phenothiazines.

Metoclopramide

Metoclopramide (10 mg orally, intramuscularly or intravenously three times a day) is an effective antiemetic whose activity closely resembles that of the phenothiazines. It acts directly on the gastrointestinal tract. Like the phenothiazines, metoclopramide can induce acute dystonic reactions and oculogyric crises. These dystonic reactions are more common in young women, and usually occur shortly after starting treatment with metoclopramide and subside within 24 hours of stopping it. Injection of an antiparkinsonian drug such as procyclidine (5–10 mg intramuscularly or intravenously) will usually stop dystonic attacks within 5–10 minutes of administration.

Metoclopramide and the phenothiazines are used as second-line treatment if the symptoms of vomiting have not resolved. Caution should be exercised when using them together in view of the combined risk of dystonic reactions.

Specific 5 hydroxytryptamine (serotonin) antagonists

Anecdotal use of this group of drugs appears to be increasing in pregnancy. No adverse effects have been found in pregnancy with the use of ondansatron, even at high doses.[36] These drugs act by blocking 5 hydroxytryptamine receptors in the gastrointestinal tract and in the central nervous system.

Corticosteroids

Corticosteroids have been used effectively as antiemetics for postoperative and carcinoma-related nausea and vomiting. Consequently, they have been introduced as treatment for nausea and vomiting in pregnancy, particularly in women who have been resistant to all other forms of pharmacological treatment. There have been several randomised controlled trials looking at the use of corticosteroids compared with placebo in women with HG, with conflicting results. While earlier studies showed benefits of corticosteroid administration (oral prednisolone or intravenous hydrocortisone),[37,38] a more recent study of 126 women found a high placebo effect and no difference in the primary outcome measure (rate of readmission), which was 34% in the group that received corticosteroids compared with 35% in the placebo group.[39]

Concerns have been expressed with regard to the safety of corticosteroids in the first trimester. Prednisolone is metabolised by the placenta and the concentration of the active compound in fetal blood is 10% of that in the mother.[40] Hydrocortisone crosses the placenta rapidly; however, most is quickly converted to inactive cortisone by fetal enzymes.[41] Studies looking at the use of corticosteroids for asthma in pregnancy have not shown any increase in congenital malformations or adverse fetal effects due to steroid therapy.[42]

Alternative treatment options

Attempts to avoid conventional pharmacological agents in pregnancy have led to studies investigating the efficacy of alternative therapies. Several trials have compared the effect of ginger with that of placebo for the treatment of nausea and vomiting in pregnancy and have reported improvement in both nausea and vomiting with the use of ginger.[43–45] However, studies examining the effect of acupuncture or acupressure compared with a sham procedure found no significant improvement in symptoms.[46]

Total parenteral and enteral nutrition

For women who are resistant to medical treatment, total parenteral nutrition may be needed to provide a means of maintaining adequate maternal nutrition. However, complications directly related to the use of total parenteral nutrition have been reported such as thrombosis, infection and metabolic disturbances.[47] Thiamine supplementation is essential when the carbohydrate-rich total parenteral nutrition is administered to reduce the risk of Wernicke's encephalopathy.

A study published in 2004 described the successful use of enteral feeding via a nasojejunal tube in women resistant to medical therapy. It showed an improvement in symptoms within 48 hours of tube insertion with resolution of symptoms after a mean of 5 days.[48]

Termination of pregnancy

In the rare situation where all other forms of therapy have failed or the condition has become life-threatening, termination of pregnancy may be the only answer.

Risk of recurrence

Women who have suffered with HG in their first pregnancy should be counselled that the risk of recurrence in the next pregnancy is approximately 15%, with the severity of the disease increasing with successive pregnancies.[49]

Conclusion

HG remains a disabling condition of unknown aetiology with potentially life-threatening complications. Until the pathogenesis of this condition can be determined, management options will be directed towards supportive treatment such as fluid replacement and vitamin supplementation and therefore will remain unsatisfactory.

References

1 Gadsby R, Barnie-Adshead A M, Jagger C. A prospective study of nausea and vomiting during pregnancy. *Br J Gen Pract* 1993;43:245–8.

2 Jewell D, Young G. Interventions for nausea and vomiting in early pregnancy. *Cochrane Database Syst Rev* 2003;(4):CD000145.

3 Fairweather D V. Nausea and vomiting in pregnancy. *Am J Obstet Gynecol* 1968;102:135–75.

4 Bailit J L. Hyperemesis gravidarium: epidemiologic findings from a large cohort. *Am J Obstet Gynecol* 2005;193:811–4.

5 Tsang I S, Katz V L, Wells S D. Maternal and fetal outcomes in hyperemesis gravidarum. *Int J Gynaecol Obstet* 1996;55:231–5.

6 Ogunyemi D A, Fong A. Hyperemesis gravidarum. *emedicine* Updated 19 June 2009 [emedicine.medscape.com/article/254751-overview].

7 Fell D B, Dodds L, Joseph K S, Allen V M, Butler B. Risk factors for hyperemesis gravidarum requiring hospital admission during pregnancy. *Obstet Gynecol* 2006;107: 277–84.

8 Danzer H, Braustein G D, Rasor J, Forsythe A, Wade M E. Maternal serum human chorionic gonadotropin concentrations and fetal sex prediction. *Fertil Steril* 1980;34:336–40.

9 Goodwin T M, Hershman J M, Cole L. Increased concentration of the free beta-subunit of human chorionic gonadotropin in hyperemesis gravidarum. *Acta Obstet Gynecol Scand* 1994;73:770–2.

10 Verberg M F, Gillott D J, Al-Fardan N, Grudzinskas J G. Hyperemesis gravidarum, a literature review. *Hum Reprod Update* 2005;11:527–39.

11 Panesar N S, Li C Y, Rogers M S. Are thyroid hormones or hCG responsible for hyperemesis gravidarum? A matched paired study in pregnant Chinese women. *Acta Obstet Gynecol Scand* 2001;80:519–24.

12 Yoshimura M, Hershman JM. Thyrotropic action of human chorionic gonadotropin. *Thyroid* 1995;5:425–34.

13 Lagiou P, Tamimi R, Mucci L A, Trichopoulos D, Adami HO, Hsieh CC. Nausea and vomiting in pregnancy in relation to prolactin, estrogens, and progesterone: a prospective study. *Obstet Gynecol* 2003;101:639–44.

14 Goodwin T M, Montoro M, Mestman J H. Transient hyperthyroidism and hyperemesis gravidarum: clinical aspects, *Am J Obstet Gynecol* 1992;167:648–52.

15 Datz F L, Christian P E, Moore J. Gender-related differences in gastric emptying. *J Nucl Med* 1987;28:1204–7.

16 Hutson W R, Roehrkasse R L, Wald A. Influence of gender and menopause on gastric emptying and motility. *Gastroenterology* 1989;96:11–7.

17 Maes B D, Spitz B, Ghoos Y F, Hiele M I, Evenepoel P, Rutgeerts P J. Gastric emptying in hyperemesis gravidarum and non-dyspeptic pregnancy. *Aliment Pharmacol Ther* 1999;13:237–43.

18 Bagis T, Gumurdulu Y, Kayaselcuk F, Yilmaz E S, Killicadag E, Tarim E. Endoscopy in hyperemesis gravidarum and Helicobacter pylori infection. *Int J Gynaecol Obstet* 2002;79:105–9.

19 Jacoby E B, Porter K B. Helicobacter pylori infection and persistent hyperemesis gravidarum. *Am J Perinatol* 1999;16:85–8.

20 FitzGerald C M. Nausea and vomiting in pregnancy. *Br J Med Psychol* 1984;57:159–65.

21 Simpson S W, Goodwin T M, Robins SB, Rizzo A A, Howes R A, Buckwalter D K, et al. Psychological factors and hyperemesis gravidarum. *J Womens Health Gend Based Med* 2001;10:471–7.

22 Johnson D R, Douglas D, Hauswald M, Tandberg D. Dehydration and orthostatic vital signs in women with hyperemesis gravidarum. *Acad Emerg Med* 1995;2:692–7.

23 Lewis G, editor. Confidential Enquiry into Maternal and Child Health. *Why Mothers Die 2000–2002. The Sixth Report of the Confidential Enquiries into Maternal Deaths in the United Kingdom.* London RCOG Press; 2004.

24 Chiossi G, Neri I, Cavazzuti M, Basso G, Facchinetti F. Hyperemesis gravidarum complicated by Wernicke encephalopathy: background, case report, and review of the literature. *Obstet Gynecol Surv* 2006;61:255–68.

25 Omer S M, al Kawi M Z, al Watban J, Bohlega S, McLean D R, Miller G. Acute Wernicke's encephalopathy associated with hyperemesis gravidarum: magnetic resonance imaging findings. *J Neuroimaging* 1995;5:251–3.

26 Castillo R A, Ray R A, Yaghmai F. Central pontine myelinolysis and pregnancy. *Obstet Gynecol* 1989;73:459–61.

27 Mazzotta P, Stewart DE, Koren G, Magee LA. Factors associated with elective termination of pregnancy among Canadian and American women with nausea and vomiting of pregnancy. *J Psychosom Obstet Gynaecol* 2001;22:7–12.

28 Swallow B L, Lindow S W, Masson E A, Hay D M. Psychological health in early pregnancy: relationship with nausea and vomiting. *J Obstet Gynaecol* 2004;24:28–32.

29 Dodds L, Fell D B, Joseph K S, Allen V M, Butler B. Outcomes of pregnancies complicated by hyperemesis gravidarum. *Obstet Gynecol* 2006;107:285–92.

30 Bashiri A, Neumann L, Maymon E, Katz M. Hyperemesis gravidarum: epidemiologic features, complications and outcome. *Eur J Obstet Gynecol Reprod Biol* 1995;63:135–8.

31 Kirk E, Papageorghiou A T, Condous G, Bottomley C, Bourne T. Hyperemesis gravidarum: is an ultrasound scan necessary? *Hum Reprod* 2006;21:2440–2.

32 Alalade AO, Khan R, Dawlatly B. Day-case management of hyperemesis gravidarum: feasibility and clinical efficacy. *J Obstet Gynaecol* 2007;27:363–4.

33 Bergin P S, Harvey P. Wernicke's encephalopathy and central pontine myelinolysis associated with hyperemesis gravidarum. *BMJ* 1992;305:517–8.

34 Koren G, Levichek Z. The teratogenicity of drugs for nausea and vomiting of pregnancy: perceived versus true risk. *Am J Obstet Gynecol* 2002;186 Suppl 5:S248–52.

35 Asker C, Norstedt Wikner B, Kallen B. Use of antiemetic drugs during pregnancy in Sweden. *Eur J Clin Pharmacol* 2005;61:899–906.

36 Tucker M L, Jackson M R, Scales M D, Spurling N W, Tweats D J, Capel-Edwards K. Ondansetron: pre-clinical safety evaluation. *Eur J Cancer Clin Oncol* 1989;25 Suppl 1:S79–S93.

37 Nelson-Piercy C, Fayers P, de Swiet M Randomised, double-blind, placebo-controlled trial of corticosteroids for the treatment of hyperemesis gravidarum, *BJOG* 2001;108:9–15.

38 Safari H R, Fassett M J, Souter I C, Alsulyman O M, Goodwin T M. The efficacy of methylprednisolone in the treatment of hyperemesis gravidarum: a randomized, double-blind, controlled study. *Am J Obstet Gynecol* 1998;179:921–4.

39 Yost N P, McIntire D D, Wians F H Jr, Ramin S M, Balko J A, Leveno K J. A randomized, placebo-controlled trial of corticosteroids for hyperemesis due to pregnancy. *Obstet Gynecol* 2003;102:1250–4.

40 Beitins I Z , Bayard F, Ances I G, Kowarski A, Migem C J. The transplacental passage of prednisone and prednisolone in pregnancy near term. *J Paediatr* 1972;81:936–45.

41 Murphy B E , Clark S J , Donald I R , Pinsky M, Vedady D. Conversion of maternal cortisol to cortisone during placental transfer to the human fetus. *Am J Obstet Gynecol* 1974;118:538–41.

42 Fitzsimons R, Greenberger P A, Patterson R. Outcome of pregnancy in women requiring corticosteroids for severe asthma. *J Allergy Clin Immunol* 1986;78:349–53.

43 Willetts K E, Ekangaki A, Eden J A. Effect of a ginger extract on pregnancy-induced nausea: a randomised controlled trial. *Aust N Z J Obstet Gynaecol* 2003;43:139–44.

44 Fischer-Rasmussen W, Kjaer S K, Dahl C, Asping U. Ginger treatment of hyperemesis gravidarum. *Eur J Obstet Gynecol Reprod Biol* 1991;38:19–24.

45 Vutyavanich T, Kraisarin T, Ruangsri R. Ginger for nausea and vomiting in pregnancy: randomized, double-masked, placebo-controlled trial. *Obstet Gynecol* 2001;97:577–82.

46 Knight B, Mudge C, Openshaw S, White A, Hart A. Effect of acupuncture on nausea of pregnancy: a randomized, controlled trial. *Obstet Gynecol* 2001;97:184–8

47 Folk J J, Leslie-Brown H F, Nosovitch J T, Silverman R K, Aubry R H. Hyperemesis gravidarum: outcomes and complications with and without total parenteral nutrition. *J Reprod Med* 2004;49:497–502.

48 Vaisman N, Kaidar R, Levin I, Lessing J B. Nasojejunal feeding in hyperemesis gravidarum – a preliminary study. *Clin Nutr* 2004;23:53–7.

49 Trogstad L I, Stoltenberg C, Magnus P, Skjaerven R, Irgens L M. Recurrence risk in hyperemesis gravidarum. *BJOG* 2005;112:1641–5.

6

Diagnosis and treatment of recurrent miscarriage

Rehan Salim

Introduction

Miscarriage is the most common complication of pregnancy, with as many as 15–20% of clinically recognised pregnancies ending in spontaneous failure.[1] The main causes of miscarriage are sporadic lethal chromosomal abnormalities and these pregnancies are destined to fail from the outset.[2,3] In fact, if all conceptions were included in the definition of miscarriage, around 40% would end in failure, with the majority occurring before the pregnancy could be clinically recognised.

However, in some couples, miscarriage can be recurrent, which is defined as three consecutive pregnancy losses before fetal viability at 24 weeks of gestation. The prevalence of this condition is approximately 1%. As the most common cause of miscarriage is aneuploidy, which is directly related to maternal age, the risk and prevalence of early pregnancy loss rises with increasing maternal age.[4] The overall prevalence of recurrent miscarriage in the population is higher than would be expected by chance alone. Statistically, the prevalence should be only 0.34%, indicating that in some couples there may be an underlying cause that puts them at higher risk. However, the calculation of the risk of three consecutive losses is based on the assumption that the baseline risk of miscarriage is 15%. This calculation does not take into account the fact that the risk of miscarriage increases with advancing maternal age. For example, the risk of miscarriage in a 40-year-old woman is at least 45% and therefore the expected prevalence of recurrent miscarriage in this age group is approximately 9%. Thus, the older the woman, the more likely the cause of her recurrent miscarriages will be embryonic aneuploidy rather than anything else.

This chapter considers the established causes of recurrent miscarriage and explores the evidence behind novel theories of pregnancy loss.

Genetic causes

Sporadic chromosomal abnormalities account for almost 70% of miscarriages and for many couples these are random, chance events. The risk of miscarriage reoccurring in these cases is not higher compared with the general population of women of similar age.[2,3] However, in around 4% of couples at least one partner will carry a chromosomal anomaly that predisposes them to miscarriage.[5] The anomaly may be in the form of a balanced translocation, where the terminal ends of two chromosomes are exchanged, or it may be a Robertsonian translocation, where there is centric fusion of two acrocentric chromosomes. The carriers of these chromosomes are phenotypically normal; however, during meiosis approximately 50–70% of gametes (and hence embryos) will inherit an unbalanced chromosomal complement that predisposes them to miscarriage.

Chromosomal translocations are identified by peripheral blood karyotype and this test should be offered to all couples presenting with recurrent first-trimester miscarriage. Those identified as carriers should be referred for genetic counselling. There is no clear consensus on the best treatment to offer these couples; however, in vitro fertilisation (IVF) with preimplantation genetic screening has been proposed by some. This procedure enables detection of chromosomally abnormal embryos with unbalanced chromosomal complements so that only chromosomally normal embryos are replaced. However, there is controversy regarding such complex treatment as the risk of miscarriage in translocation carriers is only 33% and live birth rates as high as 70% have been reported.[6]

Maternal age

Reproductive choices in society have changed over the last few decades and many women now elect to delay having children until later in life. This fact is reflected in demographic data in the UK showing that between 1985 and 2001, the number of women becoming mothers for the first time after the age of 30 years rose from 8% to 16% of all births. In keeping with this, the Human Fertilisation and Embryology Authority also reports a steady increase in the age of women presenting and undergoing fertility treatment in the UK.

Although it is important that society gives women the freedom to choose when to start their families, it takes longer for human reproductive biology to adjust to these choices. A female embryo is equipped with a cohort of oocytes that have entered meiotic arrest and remain retained within the ovaries for 10–50 years. The majority of oocytes either undergo atresia or are lost without being fertilised. Each month, a cohort of oocytes resumes development. Throughout a woman's lifetime, the healthiest oocytes are selected preferentially in young age to undergo the process of maturation and ovulation. As a result, by the end of a woman's reproductive life the majority of the oocytes retained within her ovaries are abnormal. Consistent with this, Nybo Andersen et al. have shown, in a large population-based study, that the risk of spontaneous miscarriage is directly related to maternal age and is associated with chromosomally abnormal embryos.[4] This study showed that the risk of miscarriage is 9% in 20–24-year-old women, 15% in 30–34-year-olds and 51% in 40–44-year-olds. Embryonic aneuploidy is also related to the risk of infertility. The Human Fertilisation & Embryology Authority registry data show that with advancing maternal age there is a declining prognosis for fertility treatment, so that by the age of 42 years the chance of a successful pregnancy with IVF is only 5%.

Management of maternal age as a cause of recurrent pregnancy failure remains a difficult problem. Careful counselling and information regarding the chances of success should be presented clearly to the couple. There is currently no method available to replace the oocytes that are lost earlier in life and there is nothing that can be done to improve oocyte quality.

Preimplantation genetic screening heralded much promise, as it provided a means by which only chromosomally normal embryos would be replaced in a woman who was at high risk of aneuploidy. The technique involved undergoing a cycle of intracytoplasmatic semen injection, which consists of ovarian stimulation and injection of paternal sperm into harvested oocytes. The fertilised oocytes would be allowed to develop in the laboratory for 3 days and then a single cell would be biopsied; only those embryos that were normal would then be replaced. However, many embryos demonstrated mosaicism, with up to 60% of the cells within a normal early embryo showing abnormalities on karyotyping. The cause of this phenomenon is unclear. It has been postulated that abnormal cells that are present in the early stage of human development are destined to form extraembryonic tissues (trophoblasts) rather than an embryo, or that individual abnormal cell lines undergo programmed apoptosis and regression. Therefore, many healthy embryos could have been potentially misclassified as abnormal and considered unsuitable for transfer. As a result, the pool of embryos suitable for replacement in these women was limited and often not a single healthy embryo could be found in individual cases following successful egg collection and fertilisation.

Additionally, the procedure of embryo biopsy may cause a degree of damage to the early embryo and could also reduce the chance of successful pregnancy. Twisk et al. have shown in a randomised controlled trial that screening for embryonic aneuploidy results in a significantly lower live birth rate of 24% in women receiving screening for embryonic aneuploidy compared with 35% in women undergoing conventional IVF and an odds ratio of 0.68 (95% CI 0.5–0.92) for live birth.[7]

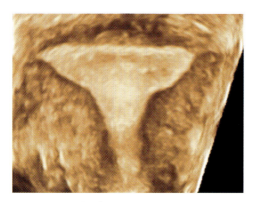

FIGURE 6.1 **A normal uterus as it appears on three-dimensional ultrasound scan**

The outer uterine contour is convex and the fundal aspect of the uterine cavity is straight.

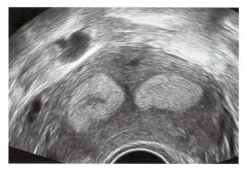

FIGURE 6.2 **Two-dimensional scan of the uterus**

On transverse view the fundal aspect of the uterine cavity appears split. This is suspicious for a major congenital anomaly but a three-dimensional scan is required to determine the nature of the abnormality.

Structural uterine abnormalities

Abnormalities of the uterus may be congenital or acquired. Congenital uterine anomalies are a range of morphological defects of uterine development that arise in early embryonic life. Their impact on reproductive failure remains a matter of controversy. At present it is believed that uterine anomalies can lead to adverse pregnancy outcomes but do not cause infertility.

In the context of recurrent miscarriage, the uterine anomaly that is classically associated with an increased risk of adverse outcomes is the septate/subseptate uterus.[8] This anomaly arises from the failure of resorption of müllerian duct tissue in the embryonic uterus with a resultant residual septum that divides the uterine cavity. It is thought either that the presence of this septum causes septal implantation or that an abnormal intrauterine environment caused by its presence can result in the loss of chromosomally normal pregnancies. The prevalence of major congenital uterine anomalies in women with recurrent miscarriage is reported as 6%; however, congenital uterine anomalies are also found in women incidentally where there is no history of recurrent pregnancy failure, with the prevalence in this latter group being around 3%.[9]

The ability of congenital uterine anomalies to cause recurrent pregnancy loss in some women and not in others has fuelled debate about their true significance. The primary reason for this was the need in the past to

TABLE 6.1 **Comparison of the severity of uterine anatomy disruption in women with an incidental diagnosis of arctuate or subseptate uterus and those with a history of recurrent miscarriage**

	Arcutate uterus			Subseptate uterus		
	Recurrent miscarriage	Low risk	P	Recurrent miscarriage	Low risk	P
Mean septum/fundal indent	5.57	5.26	>0.05	19.44	19.21	>0.05
Mean cavity length	23.72	28.71	<0.05	15.34	18.76	<0.05
Mean distortion ratio	0.19	0.15	<0.05	0.57	0.49	<0.05

use invasive tests for the diagnosis of congenital anomalies of the uterus. This precluded screening of the general population for the anomalies, so all information about their clinical significance was obtained from women with a history of infertility or recurrent miscarriage. The introduction of three-dimensional ultrasound has circumvented this issue. Studies using this technique to compare congenital uterine anomalies between low-risk women and those with a history of recurrent miscarriage showed a four-fold higher prevalence of anomalies in those who had suffered repeated pregnancy losses.[10,11] In addition, the studies showed that uterine anomalies in women with recurrent pregnancy loss tend to be more severe compared with anomalies that are diagnosed incidentally on screening (Figures 6.1–6.5 and Table 6.1).

A recent observational study investigating the severity of uterine anomalies in women with a subseptate uterus and the risk of losing a chromosomally normal embryo has shown a direct correlation, with women having a higher risk of miscarrying a normal embryo and a lower chance of live birth with increasing severity of uterine anomaly.[12]

These studies provide strong objective evidence to support the view that congenital uterine anomalies have a significant detrimental effect on women's reproductive performance. However, it is still not clear what benefits, if any, surgical correction of uterine anomalies may have on women's future reproductive performance. The evidence for current practice comes from numerous prospective observational and retrospective studies that have shown a significant improvement in the chance of a live birth after hysteroscopic metroplasty (Figure 6.6).[8]

Acquired anomalies of the uterus in the context of reproductive failure primarily include uterine fibroids and intrauterine adhesions. Fibroids are common benign tumours of the myometrium that are found in up to 40% of women by the age of 40 years. The majority of the data on the impact of uterine fibroids comes from infertile women and the pregnancies that result from fertility treatment. It is therefore difficult to say with any certainty what the true impact of uterine fibroids is on the risk of recurrent miscarriage in a spontaneously conceived pregnancy. However, several studies have shown that the

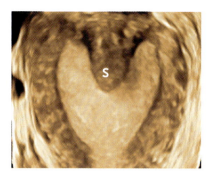

FIGURE 6.3 **Coronal three-dimensional view of the uterus showing a thick septum (S) in a case of subseptate uterus**

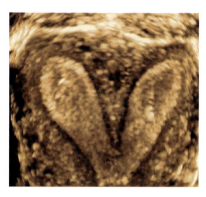

FIGURE 6.4 **Another example of a subseptate uterus**

In this case the septum is longer and thinner and is seen extending downwards almost to the level of the internal os.

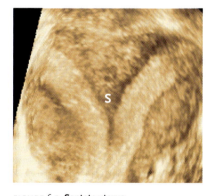

FIGURE 6.5 **Septate uterus**

Note the thin long septum extending into the cervical canal (S).

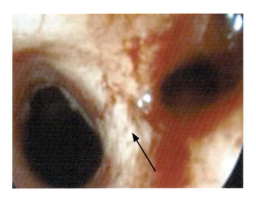

FIGURE 6.6 **Hysteroscopic view of a uterine septum (arrow) extending into the lower half of the uterine cavity**

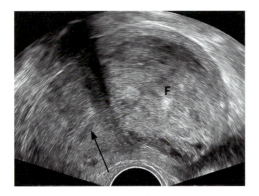

FIGURE 6.7 **Longitudinal view of the uterus**

The lower part of the cavity appears normal (arrow), while the upper part is distorted by a large submucous fibroid (F).

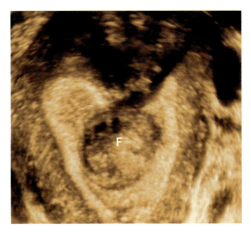

FIGURE 6.8 **Three-dimensional scan showing a submucous fibroid (F) protruding deep into the uterine cavity**

presence of a fibroid increases the risk of bleeding and spontaneous miscarriage. Benson et al. showed that, in women matched for age, the risk of spontaneous miscarriage was at least twice as high in women with fibroids than in those without, and this risk rose further in the presence of multiple fibroids.[13] This increased risk of spontaneous miscarriage would, in theory at least, increase the risk of consecutive pregnancy losses (Figures 6.7 and 6.8).

The removal of fibroids in women at increased risk of miscarriage remains controversial as well. Miscarriage rates following myomectomy have been shown to improve from 60% to 24% and from 41% to 19%.[14] However, these rates are still higher than expected, which may in part be explained by the fact that fibroids tend to be found in older women, but there remains a concern that the procedure itself may compromise the uterus to some extent and thereby increase the risk of miscarriage (Figure 6.9).[14]

The presence of intrauterine adhesions, or Asherman syndrome, is reported to increase the risk of miscarriage. In this latter situation the adhesions are usually less severe, as a greater degree of severity would lead to infertility (Figures 6.10–6.13). The spontaneous conception rate in women with Asherman syndrome is reported at 46%, with a first-trimester miscarriage rate of 40%.[15] There are very few data reporting the prevalence of intrauterine adhesions in women with recurrent miscarriage and this may in part be due to the difficulty of diagnosing this condition. Surgical correction may improve reproductive performance; however, there remains the risk of recurrence of adhesions, and all the data related to postsurgical outcomes in women with intrauterine adhesions come from infertile populations.[16]

BOX 6.1 **Clinical criteria for the diagnosis of antiphospholipid syndrome**

○ Three or more consecutive unexplained miscarriages before the 10th week of gestation.

○ One or more unexplained death of a morphologically normal fetus at 10 weeks of gestation or older.

○ One or more premature birth of a morphologically normal fetus at 34 weeks of gestation or younger associated with severe pre-eclampsia or placental insufficiency.

Antiphospholipid syndrome

The presence of maternal antibodies directed against phospholipid-binding plasma proteins, known as antiphospholipid syndrome, is a recognised treatable cause of recurrent pregnancy loss. The syndrome was originally described as the association between the presence of antiphospholipid antibodies and recurrent miscarriage, thrombosis or thrombocytopenia.[17] In contemporary practice, several clinical criteria are used to diagnose the syndrome (Box 6.1). The prevalence of these antibodies is 15% in women with recurrent miscarriage and, when left untreated, the rate of prospective pregnancy loss is 80–90%.[18]

The antiphospholipid antibodies specifically implicated in recurrent miscarriage are the lupus anticoagulant and anticardiolipin immunoglobulin G and M antibodies. The diagnosis of antiphospholipid syndrome is made when there are at least two positive results for the presence of lupus anticoagulant or the presence of anticardiolipin antibodies on tests performed at least 6 weeks apart.

Several strategies have been proposed for the treatment of antiphospholipid syndrome, including steroids, heparin, aspirin and intravenous immunoglobulins. However, only the combination of aspirin with heparin has been shown to significantly improve live birth rates and reduce the risk of miscarriage.[19]

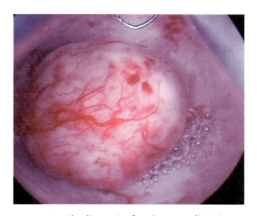

FIGURE 6.9 **The diagnosis of a submucous fibroid polyp is confirmed on hysteroscopy and the tumour is removed using a resectoscope**

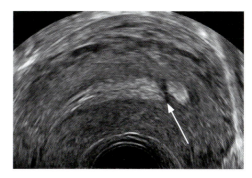

FIGURE 6.10 **A thin band of intrauterine adhesions is seen on a two-dimensional scan traversing the uterine cavity (arrow) using a resectoscope**

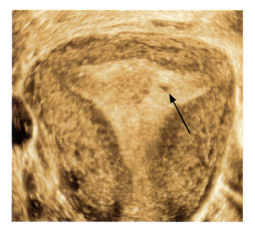

FIGURE 6.11 **The diagnosis is confirmed on a three-dimensional scan (arrow)**

Empson et al. have shown in a meta-analysis of randomised controlled trials on the use of aspirin and heparin in women with recurrent miscarriage that this combination improves the chances of a live birth to 70%.[20] The mechanism by which treatment with heparin and aspirin reduces the risk of miscarriage remains unclear; however, there is general consensus that this is most likely unrelated to any antithrombotic activity as histological analysis of miscarriage specimens does not show any increase in the presence of placental thrombosis. There is also increasing evidence to support the view that the presence of antiphospholipid antibodies impairs early trophoblast invasion and that the presence of heparin counteracts this effect.[21]

Unexplained recurrent pregnancy loss

For many couples no cause for their pregnancy failure can be identified. Although the inability to reach a diagnosis can be frustrating, it is important to consider that for these couples, with no intervention in subsequent pregnancies, the chances of live birth are around 70%.[22] Therefore, the prognosis in this latter group is good and couples should be reassured that their pregnancy loss is most likely a result of spontaneous, non-recurrent embryonic factors. However, these couples are also the most vulnerable and, in their quest for a cause for their reproductive failure, may explore novel diagnoses including immunological factors, autoantibodies, maternopaternal immune dysfunction and endometrial luteal phase dysfunction. None of these has been proved to be a cause of recurrent miscarriage and there is no proven treatment that works for these conditions (Table 6.2).

TABLE 6.2 **Summary of the investigations for recurrent miscarriage**

Investigation	Identifiable cause
Peripheral blood karyotype (both partners)	Balanced translocation
Ultrasound scan	Congenital uterine anomaly Fibroids Intrauterine adhesions
Early follicular phase follicle-stimulating hormone and estradiol	Ovarian reserve
Antiphospholipid antibodies	Lupus anticoagulant Anticardiolipin antibodies

Conclusion

Chromosomal abnormalities are the most common cause of early pregnancy loss. The risk of a pregnancy being chromosomally abnormal increases with maternal age. With an increasing number of women delaying childbirth until later in life, the number of sporadic and recurrent miscarriages is also likely to increase. However, all women with a history of recurrent pregnancy loss should be offered testing to detect and treat any gynaecological and systemic abnormalities that are associated with an increased risk of early pregnancy loss. The value of various interventions for reducing the risk of miscarriage, however, is controversial as only a few of them have been examined adequately in well-conducted prospective randomised trials.

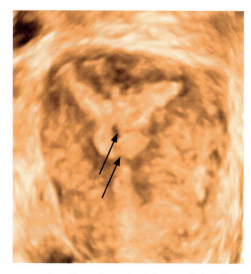

FIGURE 6.12 **Three-dimensional ultrasound view of the uterine cavity in a woman with severe intrauterine adhesions**

The uterine cavity is grossly distorted with bands of adhesions at the level of the internal os and in the centre of the cavity (arrows).

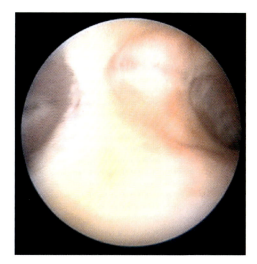

FIGURE 6.13 **Hysteroscopic view of intrauterine adhesions affecting the upper central part of the uterine cavity**

Courtesy of Mr Ertan Saridogan, University College Hospital, London.

References

1 Chard T. Frequency of implantation and early pregnancy loss in natural cycles. *Baillieres Clin Obstet Gynaecol* 1991;5:179–89.

2 Stephenson M D, Awartani K A, Robinson W P. Cytogenetic analysis of miscarriages from couples with recurrent miscarriage: a case–control study. *Hum Reprod* 2002;17:446–51.

3 Hogge W A, Byrnes A L, Lanasa M C, Surti U. The clinical use of karyotyping spontaneous abortions. *Am J Obstet Gynecol* 2003;189:397–400.

4 Nybo Andersen A M, Wohlfahrt J, Christens P, Olsen J, Melbye M. Maternal age and fetal loss: population based register linkage study. *BMJ* 2000;320:1708–12.

5 Clifford K, Rai R, Watson H, Regan L. An informative protocol for the investigation of recurrent miscarriage: preliminary experience of 500 consecutive cases. *Hum Reprod* 1994;9:1328–32.

6 Stephenson M D, Sierra S. Reproductive outcomes in recurrent pregnancy loss associated with a parental carrier of a structural chromosome rearrangement. *Hum Reprod* 2006;21:1076–82.

7 Twisk M, Mastenbroek S, Hoek A, Heineman M J, van der Veen F, Bossuyt P M, et al. No beneficial effect of preimplantation genetic screening in women of advanced maternal age with a high risk for embryonic aneuploidy. *Hum Reprod* 2008;23:2813–7.

8 Homer H A, Li TC, Cooke I D. The septate uterus: a review of management and reproductive outcome. *Fertil Steril* 2000;73:1–14.

9 Infertility revisited: the state of the art today and tomorrow. The ESHRE Capri Workshop. European Society for Human Reproduction and Embryology. *Hum Reprod* 1996;11:1779–807.

10 Salim R, Regan L, Woelfer B, Backos M, Jurkovic D. A comparative study of the morphology of congenital uterine anomalies in women with and without a history of recurrent first trimester miscarriage. *Hum Reprod* 2003;18:162–6.

11 Salim R, Woelfer B, Backos M, Regan L, Jurkovic D. Reproducibility of three-dimensional ultrasound diagnosis of congenital uterine anomalies. *Ultrasound Obstet Gynecol* 2003;21:578–82.

12 Sugiura-Ogasawara M, Ozaki Y, Kitaori T, Kumagai K, Suzuki S. Midline uterine defect size is correlated with miscarriage of euploid embryos in recurrent cases. *Fertil Steril* 2010;93:1983–8.

13 Benson C B, Chow J S, Chang-Lee W. Outcome of pregnancies in women with uterine leiomyomas identified by sonography in the first trimester. *J Clin Ultrasound* 2001;29:261–4.

14 Li T C, Mortimer R, Cooke I D. Myomectomy: a retrospective study to examine reproductive performance before and after surgery. *Hum Reprod* 1999;14:1735–40.

15 Schenker J G, Margoliath E J. Intrauterine adhesions: an updated appraisal. *Fertil Steril* 1982;37:593–610.

16 Berman J M. Intrauterine adhesions. *Semin Reprod Med* 2008;26:349–55.

17 Harris E N. Syndrome of the black swan. *Br J Rheumatol* 1987;26:324–6.

18 Rai R S, Clifford K, Cohen H, Regan L. High prospective fetal loss rate in untreated pregnancies of women with recurrent miscarriage and antiphospholipid antibodies. *Hum Reprod* 1995;10:3301–4.

19 Rai R, Cohen H, Dave M, Regan L. Randomised controlled trial of aspirin and aspirin plus heparin in pregnant women with recurrent miscarriage associated with phospholipid antibodies (or antiphospholipid antibodies). *BMJ* 1997;314:253–7.

20 Empson M, Lassere M, Craig J C, Scott J R. Recurrent pregnancy loss with antiphospholipid antibody: a systematic review of therapeutic trials. *Obstet Gynecol* 2002;99:135–44.

21 Rai R, Regan L. Recurrent miscarriage. *Lancet* 2006;368:601–11.

22 Rai R, Clifford K, Regan L. The modern preventative treatment of recurrent miscarriage. *Br J Obstet Gynaecol* 1996;103:106–10.

7 Differential diagnosis and management of molar pregnancy

Eric Jauniaux

Introduction

Molar pregnancies result from disorders of human fertilisation. They are the most common form of gestational trophoblastic disease, which incorporates a wide spectrum of abnormalities of trophoblastic development. Hydatidiform moles were first described by Hippocrates in ancient Greece. The etymology is probably derived from the Greek word *hydatis* meaning 'a drop of water', referring to the watery content of the cysts, and the Persian word *mylon* meaning a misshapen thing (false conception). The modern medical term hydatidiform mole refers to a disorder of placental development in which the villous mesenchyme, vasculature and trophoblast are all affected and there is little or no fetal development.

Molar pregnancies are characterised by villous hydrops. Trophoblastic hyperplasia is the characteristic microscopic feature of true molar pregnancies.[1–6] Biochemical analysis of the fluid from molar vesicles indicates that it is derived from the diffusion of maternal plasma but also contains specific trophoblastic proteins. These biochemical findings suggest that the hydropic (hydatidiform) transformation of the villous mesenchyme is caused by maldevelopment, regression or lack of the villous vasculature, which compromises the drainage of fluid produced by the trophoblast.[7] Mild to moderate generalised villous oedema, which is often found following the demise of an embryo or early fetus, supports this concept and highlights the fact that hydropic villous changes are not exclusive to molar pregnancies. Hydatidiform transformation of villi is a non-specific feature of vascular dysfunction and only the hyperplastic microscopic appearance of the trophoblast is decisive for the diagnosis of molar pregnancy. Hyperplasia can be identified histologically before the hydropic villous changes are visible macroscopically.

The distinction between complete hydatidiform moles (CHM) and partial hydatidiform moles (PHM) was first made in the late 1970s on the basis of gross morphological, histological and cytogenetic criteria.[1,2] The clinical and pathological picture of the two molar syndromes overlaps to a degree[3,4] since the phenotype and natural history of PHM seem to represent milder versions

TABLE 7.1 **Comparison of the incidence of the main semiological features in complete (CHM) and partial hydatidiform moles (PHM) diagnosed during the second semester of pregnancy**

	Incidence	
Symptoms	CHM %	PHM %
Vaginal bleeding	60	4
Uterine enlargement	25	10
Hyperemesis	10	Rare
Anaemia	5	Exceptional
Multicystic ovaries	10–20	Rare
Pre-eclampsia	1–2	2.5

of those seen in cases of CHM (Table 7.1). The estimated incidence of PHM is 1/700 pregnancies whereas the incidence of CHM is around 1/1500–2000 pregnancies.[4-6]

The vast majority of complete and partial moles miscarry spontaneously during the first 3–4 months of pregnancy. The estimated incidence of molar placenta is 1/41 miscarriages.[8,9] Although these data are not population-based, they suggest that most women presenting with a molar pregnancy are likely to be first seen in an early pregnancy unit and an accurate diagnosis is thus essential for optimal management. With the introduction of high-resolution transvaginal ultrasound scanning, very few women with a CHM should present beyond the first trimester. Diagnosing women with early molar pregnancy is important to plan appropriate surgical evacuation, assess the risk of major haemorrhage and identify women at risk of developing persistent trophoblastic disease.

The various forms of molar pregnancy have different epidemiological, genetic and pathological features, which facilitates early preoperative diagnosis in the first trimester of pregnancy. The main focus of this chapter is the differential diagnosis and management of molar gestations in early pregnancy.

Diagnosis

Ultrasound and serum human chorionic gonadotrophin

The prevalence of the different types of gestational trophoblastic disease in the first trimester of pregnancy is unknown. Vaginal bleeding is the most common presenting symptom in the majority of women diagnosed with CHM.

These women experience bleeding in early pregnancy and are often referred to an early pregnancy unit for an ultrasound examination in the first trimester. However, bleeding occurs less commonly in cases of PHM (Table 7.1). In the majority of cases the main aim of ultrasound examination is to differentiate between uncomplicated miscarriage and molar pregnancy.

Abdominal ultrasound examination of the placenta should correctly identify vesicular villi by the end of the first trimester.[4] Molar ultrasound features in CHM typically reveal a uterine cavity filled with multiple sonolucent areas (Figure 7.1) of varying size and shape

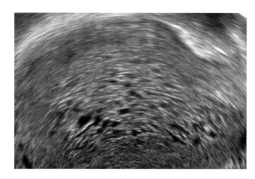

FIGURE 7.1 **Complete hydatidiform mole at 14 weeks of gestation**

('snowstorm' appearance) without any associated embryonic or fetal structures (Table 7.2). Large sonolucent areas or maternal lakes, which are often found in CHM, are caused by stasis of maternal blood between the molar villi. Before 12 weeks of gestation some partial moles may present as an enlarged

TABLE 7.2 **Ultrasound differential diagnosis of molar pregnancy in early pregnancy**

Category	Ultrasound features
Complete hydatidiform mole	
Single	○ Avascular snowstorm appearance ○ No fetus ○ Multicystic ovaries (20%)
Multiple pregnancy	○ Avascular snowstorm appearance ○ Normal fetus with normal placenta ○ Multicystic ovaries (>50%)
Partial hydatidiform mole	
Continuing pregnancy	○ Swiss cheese appearance/placentomegaly ○ Small crown–rump length (<10th percentile) ○ Fetal malformations
Miscarriage	○ Transverse to anteroposterior gestational sac diameter ratio >1.5 ○ Cystic changes in the placenta ○ Increased placental echogenicity ○ Fetal remnants
Pseudomole	
Mesenchymal dysplasia	○ Swiss cheese appearance/placentomegaly ○ Normal fetal anatomy and growth ○ Fetal malformations and macrosomy if part of Beckwith–Weidemann syndrome
Trisomy/monosomy	○ Swiss cheese appearance ○ Fetal malformations

placenta without or with only a few vesicular changes on both transabdominal and transvaginal ultrasound examination. Theca-lutein cysts secondary to the very high human chorionic gonadotrophin (hCG) levels may be diagnosed in up to 20% of CHM cases and produce enlarged ovaries with either a 'soap bubble' or a 'spoke wheel' appearance. The role of Doppler ultrasound is limited in both types of mole: in CHM it almost always demonstrates high velocities and low resistance to flow in the uterine arterial circulation and will be of clinical interest only in the diagnosis of an invasive mole.

Complete hydatidiform moles

CHM are almost always diploid, with their chromosomes totally derived from the paternal genome as a result of endoreduplication (duplication without cell cytokinesis) after monospermic fertilisation or, more rarely, dispermic fertilisation of an anucleate oocyte (devoid of the maternal X,23).[10] This entirely androgenic conceptus is characterised by generalised trophoblastic hyperplasia and rapidly developing villous oedema with central cistern formation, giving the placenta a macroscopic appearance of a 'bunch of grapes'.[1-4]

The prevalence of CHM varies geographically from 1/200 pregnancies in China to 1/1500 pregnancies in Europe and North America.[11-13] Maternal age less than 20 and over 35 years are the best established risk factors for CHM.[14] CHM can also develop in 30 000–100 000 pregnancies as part of a multiple gestation[15] and, exceptionally, in postmenopausal women.[16,17]

Classically, women with CHM present with vaginal bleeding, uterine enlargement greater than expected for gestational age and abnormally high levels of serum hCG. Maternal complications can include pregnancy-induced hypertension, hyperthyroidism, hyperemesis, anaemia and the development of ovarian theca-lutein cysts in patients with marked hCG elevations as a result of ovarian hyperstimulation (Table 7.1).

With routine use of high-resolution ultrasound in the first trimester of pregnancy, the incidence of all these complications has decreased over the last 20 years.[4-6,18-22] Vaginal bleeding remains the most common presenting symptom and is seen in approximately 90% of cases; other classic signs and symptoms such as excessive uterine enlargement, theca-lutein cysts, hyperemesis, pre-eclampsia, hyperthyroidism and respiratory insufficiency are less commonly seen.[12] Ultrasound diagnosis of CHM is usually possible before 12 weeks of gestation[22-29] (Table 7.3). Data comparing ultrasound and histological features indicate that at least 80% of CHM should be diagnosed at the time of the first ultrasound examination.[29] Data also indicate that CHM are associated with maternal serum hCG levels ranging between 10 and 200 multiples of the median and that maternal serum beta-hCG can help in the differ-

TABLE 7.3 **Comparison of ultrasound mean gestational age at diagnosis and detection rate of complete and partial hydatidiform moles in retrospective studies**

Author	CHM			PHM		
	n	GA (weeks)	DR (%)	n	GA (weeks)	DR (%)
Lindholm[23]	75	12.4	84	60	14.3	30
Lazarus[24]	21	10.5	57	–	–	–
Benson[25]	24	8.7	71	–	–	–
Fowler[26]	200	10.0	79	178	10.0	29
Kirk[27]	20	–	95	41	–	20

CHM = complete hydatidiform mole | DR = detection rate | GA = gestational age | PHM = partial hydatidiform mole.

ential diagnosis among early CHM, missed miscarriages and uterine tumours. Ovarian dysgerminomas, which are the most frequent malignant germ cell tumours in women, may spread to the uterus and appear as a heterogeneous intrauterine mass with multiple echolucent spaces.[20] Uterine tumours such as sarcomas or lymphomas may also have features similar to those of a CHM on ultrasound and should theoretically be considered in the differential diagnosis.[22] These tumours do not usually produce placentofetal hormonal markers such as hCG or alphafetoprotein.

A CHM may co-exist with a normal fetus and its placenta if there is molar transformation of one ovum in a dizygotic twin pregnancy.[15] Before the use of ultrasound for the screening of trisomy 21 at 11–14 weeks of gestation, these rare cases were often only diagnosed at around 18–20 weeks, which is later in gestation than would be expected in cases of singleton CHM. One study found that, as a CHM produces such a characteristic vesicular sonographic pattern (Figure 7.2), their association with a normal gestational sac can be accurately determined from 11 weeks of gestation.[15,30] Earlier in pregnancy, these are often misdiagnosed as a degenerating fibroid or a subchorionic haematoma. This study also found that at 11–14 weeks of gestation these cases present with maternal serum beta-hCG levels over 100 multiples of the median and thus hCG level is a useful adjunct in early differential diagnosis and follow-up in cases of conservative management.[29,31]

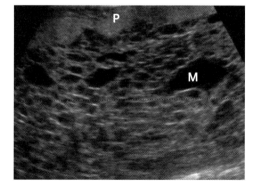

FIGURE 7.2 **Complete hydatidiform mole (M) associated with a normal pregnancy with a normal placenta (P) at 22 weeks of gestation**

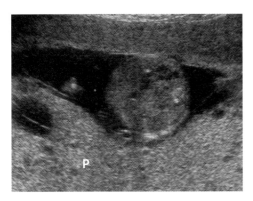

FIGURE 7.3 **Triploid partial hydatidiform mole type I (paternally derived, i.e. diandric triploidy) at 17 weeks of gestation**

Note that the placenta (P) is enlarged and contains molar villi.

Partial hydatidiform moles

The term PHM refers to the combination of a fetus with a placenta containing localised villous molar degenerations. Histologically, PHM is characterised by focal swelling of the villous tissue and focal trophoblastic hyperplasia in the presence of an embryo or fetus.[1-4,32] The abnormal villi are scattered within macroscopically normal placental tissue that tends to retain its shape. The hydatidiform changes are usually focal, resulting in an irregular patchwork of seemingly normal and abnormal areas (Figure 7.3). The histopathological definition of PHM applies only when the villous hydatidiform changes are associated with trophoblastic hyperplasia, which, similar to cases of CHM, cannot be detected by ultrasound.

The estimated incidence of PHM is 1/700 pregnancies and does not seem to vary significantly around the world.[1,4,8,12] Partial moles are triploid in about 90% of cases, having inherited two sets of chromosomes from the father and one from the mother.[1-4] Two fetal phenotypes have been delineated: type I (paternally derived, i.e. diandric triploidy), where the fetus is relatively well grown, has a proportionate head size and presents with placental partial molar changes (Figure 7.3), and type II (maternally derived, i.e. digynic triploidy), where the fetus presents with severe asymmetrical growth restriction and a placenta that is not associated with any hydatidiform changes.[3,4,10,33]

Women with PHM generally present with signs and symptoms consistent with early embryonic demise or incomplete miscarriage. In most cases the diagnosis of PHM is made on histological review of uterine curettings.[29,32] The classic presentation described for CHM is rare in cases of PHM (Table 7.1) and there have been only a few isolated case reports of PHM associated with early severe pregnancy-induced hypertension and hyperthyroidism.[34,35] Triploidies are lethal chromosomal abnormalities and most embryos affected by this defect are miscarried within a few weeks following conception.[4,32] Genetic studies have shown that most triploid miscarriages are diandric. Digynic triploid fetuses without major congenital anomalies may progress beyond the first trimester only to be detected on a detailed ultrasound examination at 20 weeks of gestation.[33]

When the ratio of the transverse to anteroposterior dimensions of the gestational sac is greater than 1.5 and the placenta contains obvious focal cystic changes, the predictive value of ultrasound diagnosis of PHM in early pregnancy is around 90%.[12] In PHM, the hydatidiform transformation develops more slowly than in CHM and before 12 weeks of gestation many cases present simply as an enlarged placenta without obvious macroscopic vesicular changes.[19,21,29,33] It is therefore not surprising that the ultrasound diagnosis of PHM is less accurate than that of CHM at the same gestational age and that around 70% of cases are missed during the first trimester (Table 7.3).[29,36–38] Several ultrasound features have been identified that facilitate the early ultrasound detection of molar change in cases of first-trimester early embryonic demise. These include distorted gestational sac diameter ratios, cystic changes and increased echogenicity of placental tissue at the maternal–embryonic interface.[22,23,29,36–38] Pre-evacuation maternal serum hCG levels may be a useful adjunct to histological diagnosis of PHM in first-trimester spontaneous miscarriages, in particular in cases with unusual ultrasound appearances. In a prospective preliminary study, nine of 13 (69%) molar pregnancies in which a preoperative maternal serum hCG was available demonstrated an hCG of 2.0–10.8 multiples of the median.[29] In continuing pregnancies the fetus almost always presents with severe growth restriction and various structural abnormalities.[4]

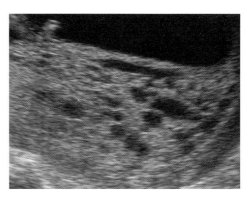

FIGURE 7.4 **Pseudomole in a case of mesenchymal dysplasia at 20 weeks of gestation**

Villous hydatidiform transformation can be found in association with tetraploidy and other polyploid chromosomal abnormalities.[4] As the vast majority of tetraplodies miscarry spontaneously during the first weeks of pregnancy, partial 'molar' placentas resulting from a double or triple paternal contribution have been rarely described in continuing pregnancies. Confined placental diploid or triploid mosaicism may appear as a triploid partial mole on scan, but in these cases the fetus is anatomically normal and has a diploid karyotype.[4,10] Ultrasound and pathological examination may in rare cases be complicated by the fact that the molar placental tissue comes from a reabsorbed vanishing twin. In these cases the mother remains at risk of developing complications of triploid PHM and in particular she may subsequently develop early pre-eclampsia and persistent trophoblastic disease.

Pseudomoles

Although there is a well-established histopathological association between molar changes of the villi and trophoblastic hyperplasia, hydropic villous changes can be found in conditions unrelated to gestational trophoblastic disease such as mesenchymal dysplasia (Figure 7.4). The prenatal diagnosis of mesenchymal dysplasia was first reported in 1991 and can be found as part of the Beckwith–Wiedemann syndrome.[4,39] An association between benign molar changes without trophoblastic hyperplasia and trisomy 13 has also been described.[40] There are now more than 65 cases of mesenchymal dysplasia (hyperplasia) and several case reports of trisomy 13 presenting as a PHM.[39–43] A case report[44] describing a case of trisomy 13 presenting as a PHM but showing histological changes similar to those found in mesenchymal dysplasia supports the hypothesis of a vascular malformation of the stem villi[40] as the main pathophysiological basis for the changes found in the mesenchyme of the placenta in these cases.

Cases of mesenchymal dysplasia have been diagnosed from the end of the first trimester.[20,39] In cases of early embryonic demise (before 7–8 weeks of menstrual age), with or without a chromosomal abnormality, the progressive disappearance of the villous vasculature after embryonic death leads to villous hydrops; however, this does not herald a true PHM.[4,22,29] Focal villous hydropic changes may also be found in pregnancies presenting with monosomy X and are probably also caused by insufficient development of the villous vasculature or by villous degeneration in some placental areas.[4]

Histological diagnosis

Histological diagnosis of CHM can be difficult because the molar changes may be obscured by necrosis due to prolonged retention in utero. In addition, not all pathologists are sufficiently trained to make a confident diagnosis of CHM. In the UK, histological specimens suggestive of molar pregnancy are reviewed by an expert pathology team in a tertiary referral centre to confirm the diagnosis.

Even in expert hands, the diagnosis of molar changes, particularly in PHM, can be difficult.[32,45–47] Karyotyping or ploidy determination is helpful in difficult cases, but these techniques are not used as the first-line diagnostic tools because they are expensive and time-consuming. DNA ploidy assessment can be useful in some cases to discriminate between PHM and CHM and is cheaper and faster than karyotyping.[45,47] However, the test is not perfect and it may lead to misclassification in cases of contamination with maternal tissues. In addition, ploidy analysis cannot distinguish between a diploid molar pregnancy and hydropic abortion. Differences in expression of imprinted genes between CHM and PHM pregnancies have been shown to be useful in differential diagnosis.[48] Using immunohistochemical techniques, the expression of a known imprinted gene can be used to indicate the presence of a functional maternal copy of that gene in PHM and the absence of the maternal copy in CHM.[49] Recent studies have also demonstrated the use of p57 immunostaining and molecular genotyping for improving diagnosis of molar pregnancies.[50]

Management

Following uterine evacuation, 10–20% of women with a CHM develop a gestational trophoblastic neoplasia and will require chemotherapy.[5,6,11,12] The gestational trophoblastic neoplasias include mainly persistent trophoblastic disease, while choriocarcinoma accounts for 1–2% of cases. The reported risk of persistent trophoblastic disease following the uterine evacuation of a persistent trophoblastic disease is variable, with rates ranging between 0.1% and 11%.[5,6,11,12,44,51,52] Some of this variation is probably the result of differences between population-based versus specialist centre-based series data. Wide variation in the prevalence of persistent trophoblastic disease after PHM is also probably due to the absence of epidemiological data from large unselected populations and variations in the quality of histological examination. True choriocarcinoma is rare after PHM but a few cases have recently been reported.[53,54] Very young age (under 20 years) and older age (over 40 years) and a history of previous molar pregnancy are associated with the development of persistent trophoblastic disease.[6,12]

Suction curettage under continuous ultrasound guidance is the preferred method of evacuation regardless of uterine size in women who desire to preserve fertility. Medical termination of molar pregnancies, including cervical preparation prior to surgical evacuation, should be avoided owing to the risk of dissemination of trophoblastic tissue through the uterine venous circulation. Brisk bleeding sometimes occurs during cervical dilatation due to the passage of blood retained within the uterine cavity. Uterotonics such as oxytocin and/or misoprostol should be withheld until the evacuation is complete, if at all possible. In suspected cases of molar pregnancies on ultrasound scan, serum hCG measurements can be used to minimise the risk of false negative diagnosis.[29]

Following evacuation of products of conception, all women with a diagnosis of a molar pregnancy should be referred to a specialist centre and followed up with serial hCG measurements to ensure remission.[5,6] Protocols may vary between different countries, but in general patients should have regular (weekly) measurement of serum and urine hCG levels for 6 weeks until levels are undetectable, and then monthly for 6 months.[55–57] Effective contraception is essential during the entire follow-up period to ensure reliable monitoring of hCG concentrations. Although data from other countries suggest that the combined oral contraceptive pill may be safe to use, in the UK it is advised that it should not be prescribed to women whose hCG levels remain high. Women should be advised to avoid becoming pregnant for 6 months after hCG levels have returned to normal.

All women with a histological diagnosis of molar pregnancy in the UK should be registered with one of three centres: Ninewells Hospital (Dundee), Weston Park Hospital (Sheffield) or Charing Cross Hospital (London).[5] In a review by the New England Trophoblastic Disease Center, none of the women with hCG levels under 5 units/l developed persistent trophoblastic disease.[6,12] If pathological review is unavailable, hCG should be measured 3–4 weeks after termination to identify women with persistently raised values who need to be followed up.

Conclusion

Molar pregnancies represent a relatively rare complication of pregnancy. They typically present with first-trimester bleeding and clinical staff in early pregnancy units should be familiar with their clinical symptoms and typical ultrasound features. An accurate early diagnosis facilitates optimal management and timely referral to the regional trophoblastic disease centre for further follow-up.

References

1 Szulman A E, Surti U. The syndromes of hydatidiform mole. I. Cytogenetic and morphologic correlations. *Am J Obstet Gynecol* 1978;131:665–71.

2 Szulman A E, Surti U. The syndromes of hydatidiform mole. II. Morphologic evolution of complete and partial mole. *Am J Obstet Gynecol* 1978;132:20–7.

3 Szulman A E, Surti U. The clinicopathologic profile of the partial hydatidiform mole. *Obstet Gynecol* 1982;59:597–602.

4 Jauniaux E. Partial moles: from postnatal to prenatal diagnosis. *Placenta* 1999;20:379–88.

5 Sebire N J, Seckl M J. Gestational trophoblastic disease: current management of hydatidiform mole. *BMJ* 2008;337:a1193.

6 Berkowitz R S, Goldstein D P. Clinical practice. Molar pregnancy. *N Engl J Med* 2009;360:1639–45.

7 Jauniaux E, Gulbis B, Hyett J, Nicolaides K H. Biochemical analyses of mesenchymal fluid in early pregnancy. *Am J Obstet Gynecol* 1998;178:765–9.

8 Jeffers M D, O'Dwyer P, Curran B, Leader M, Gillan J E. Partial hydatidiform mole: a common but underdiagnosed condition. A 3-year retrospective clinicopathological and DNA flow cytometric analysis. *Int J Gynecol Pathol* 1993;12:315–23.

9 Fukunaga M. Early partial hydatidiform mole: prevalence, histopathology, DNA ploidy, and persistence rate. *Virchows Arch* 2000;437:180–4.

10 Devrientd K. Hydatidiform mole and triploidy: the role of genomic imprinting in placental development. *Hum Reprod Update* 2005;11:137–42.

11 Palmer J R. Advances in the epidemiology of gestational trophoblastic disease. *J Reprod Med* 1994;39:155–62.

12 Berkowitz R S, Goldstein DP. Current management of gestational trophoblastic diseases. *Gynecol Oncol* 2009;112:654–62.

13 Shi Y F, Li J Q, Zheng W, Chen X J, Qiao Y H, Hao M, et al. Survey of gestational trophoblastic disease incidence among 3.6 million pregnancies in China. *Zhonghua Fu Chan Ke Za Zhi* 2005;40:76–8.

14 Altman A D, Bentley B, Murray S, Bentley J R. Maternal age-related rates of gestational trophoblastic disease. *Obstet Gynecol* 2008;112:244–50.

15 Wee L, Jauniaux E. Prenatal diagnosis and management of twin pregnancies complicated by a co-existing molar pregnancy. *Prenat Diagn* 2005;25:772–6.

16 Abike F, Temizkan O, Payasli A, Avsar F, Karahan N, Baspinar S. Postmenopausal complete hydatidiform mole: a case report. *Maturitas* 2008;59:95–8.

17 Camuzcuoglu H, Toy H, Camuzcuoglu A, Ozalp S S. Complete mole hydatidiform in a postmenopausal woman. *Eur J Obstet Gynecol Reprod Biol* 2009;142:85–6.

18 Mangili G, Garavaglia E, Cavoretto P, Gentile C, Scarfone G, Rabaiotti E. Clinical presentation of hydatidiform mole in northern Italy: has it changed in the last 20 years? *Am J Obstet Gynecol* 2008;198:302.e1–4.

19 Hou J L, Wan X R, Xiang Y, Qi Q W, Yang X Y. Changes of clinical features in hydatidiform mole: analysis of 113 cases. *J Reprod Med* 2008;53:629–33.

20 Jauniaux E, Nicolaides K H. Early ultrasound diagnosis and follow-up of molar pregnancies. *Ultrasound Obstet Gynecol* 1997;9:17–21.

21 Kerkmeijer L G, Massuger L F, Ten Kate-Booij M J, Sweep FC, Thomas CM. Earlier diagnosis and serum human chorionic gonadotropin regression in complete hydatidiform moles. *Obstet Gynecol* 2009;113:326–31.

22 Jauniaux E. Ultrasound diagnosis and follow-up of gestational trophoblastic disease. *Ultrasound Obstet Gynecol* 1998;11:367–77.

23 Lindholm H, Flam F. The diagnosis of molar pregnancy by sonography and gross morphology. *Acta Obstet Gynecol Scand* 1999;78:6–9.

24 Lazarus E, Hulka C, Siewert B, Levine D. Sonographic appearance of early complete molar pregnancies. *J Ultrasound Med* 1999;18:589–93.

25 Benson C B, Genest D R, Bernstein M R, Soto-Wright V, Goldstein DP, Berkowitz RS. Sonographic appearance of first trimester complete hydatidiform moles. *Ultrasound Obstet Gynecol* 2000;16:188–91.

26 Fowler D J, Lindsay I, Seckl M J, Sebire N J. Routine pre-evacuation ultrasound diagnosis of hydatidiform mole: experience of more than 1000 cases from a regional referral center. *Ultrasound Obstet Gynecol* 2006;27:56–60.

27 Kirk E, Papageorghiou A T, Condous G, Bottomley C, Bourne T. The accuracy of first trimester ultrasound in the diagnosis of hydatidiform mole. *Ultrasound Obstet Gynecol* 2007;29:70–5.

28 Fowler D J, Lindsay I, Seckl M J, Sebire N J. Histomorphometric features of hydatidiform moles in early pregnancy: relationship to detectability by ultrasound examination. *Ultrasound Obstet Gynecol* 2007;29:76–80.

29 Johns J, Greenwold N, Buckley S, Jauniaux E. A prospective study of ultrasound screening for molar pregnancies in missed miscarriages. *Ultrasound Obstet Gynecol* 2005;25:493–7.

30 Jauniaux E, Sebire N. Placental and fetal malignancies. In: Kehoe S, Jauniaux E, Martin-Hirsch P, Savage P, editors. *Cancer and Reproductive Health*. London: RCOG Press; 2008. p. 187–204.

31 Jauniaux E, Bersinger N A, Gulbis B, Meuris S. The contribution of maternal serum markers in the early prenatal diagnosis of molar pregnancies. *Hum Reprod* 1999;14;842–6.

32 Jauniaux E, Kadri R, Hustin J. Partial mole and triploidy: screening patients with first-trimester spontaneous abortion. *Obstet Gynecol* 1996;88:616–9.

33 Zaragoza M V, Surti U, Redline R W, Millie E, Chakravarti A, Hassold T J. Parental origin and phenotype of triploidy in spontaneous abortions: predominance of diandry and association with the partial hydatidiform mole. *Am J Hum Genet* 2000;66:1807–20.

34 Falkert A, Yildiz A, Seelbach-Goebel B. Partial mole with fetal triploidy as a cause for imminent HELLP-syndrome at 16 weeks of gestation. *Arch Gynecol Obstet* 2009;279:423–5.

35 Chiniwala N U, Woolf P D, Bruno C P, Kaur S, Spector H, Yacono K. Thyroid storm caused by a partial hydatidiform mole. *Thyroid* 2008;18:479–81.

36 Jauniaux E, Brown R, Snijders R J, Noble P, Nicolaides K H. Early prenatal diagnosis of triploidy. *Am J Obstet Gynecol* 1997;176:550–4.

37 Naumoff P, Szulman A E, Weinstein B, Mazer J, Surti U. Ultrasonography of partial hydatidiform mole. *Radiology* 1981;140:467–70.

38 Fine C, Bundy A L, Berkowitz R S, Boswell S B, Berezin A F, Doubilet PM. Sonographic diagnosis of partial hydatidiform mole. *Obstet Gynecol* 1989;73:414–18.

39 Jauniaux E, Nicolaides K H, Hustin J. Perinatal features associated with placental mesenchymal dysplasia. *Placenta* 1997;18:701–6.

40 Jauniaux E, Hadler A, Partington C. A case of partial mole associated with trisomy 13. *Ultrasound Obstet Gynecol* 1998;11:62–4.

41 Ang D C, Rodríguez Urrego P A, Prasad V. Placental mesenchymal dysplasia: a potential misdiagnosed entity. *Arch Gynecol Obstet* 2009;279:937–9.

42 Chen C P. Placental abnormalities and preeclampsia in trisomy 13 pregnancies. *Taiwan J Obstet Gynecol* 2009;48:3–8.

43 Müngen E, Dundar O, Muhcu M, Haholu A, Tunca Y. Placental mesenchymal dysplasia associated with trisomy 13: sonographic findings. *J Clin Ultrasound* 2008;36:454–6.

44 Wielsma S, Kerkmeijer L, Bekkers R, Pyman J, Tan J, Quinn M. Persistent trophoblast disease following partial molar pregnancy. *Aust N Z J Obstet Gynaecol* 2006;46:119–23.

45 Genest DR. Partial hydatidiform mole: clinicopathological features, differential diagnosis, ploidy and molecular studies, and gold standards for diagnosis. *Int J Gynecol Pathol* 2001;20:315–22.

46 Deavers M T, Kalhor N, Silva EG. Diagnostic problems with trophoblastic lesions. *Arch Pathol Lab Med* 2008;132:168–74.

47 Niemann I, Hansen E S, Sunde L. The risk of persistent trophoblastic disease after hydatidiform mole classified by morphology and ploidy. *Gynecol Oncol* 2007;104:411–5.

48 Bell K A, Van Deerlin V, Addya K, Clevenger C V, Van Deerlin P G, Leonard D G. Molecular genetic testing from paraffin-embedded tissue distinguishes nonmolar hydropic abortion from hydatidiform mole. *Mol Diagn* 1999;4:11–9.

49 Thaker H M, Berlin A, Tycko B, Goldstein D P, Berkowitz RS, Castrillon DH, et al. Immunohistochemistry for the imprinted gene product IPL/PHLDA2 for facilitating the differential diagnosis of complete hydatidiform mole. *J Reprod Med* 2004;49:630–6.

50 McConnell T G, Murphy K M, Hafez M, Vang R, Ronnett BM. Diagnosis and subclassification of hydatidiform moles using p57 immunohistochemistry and molecular genotyping: validation and prospective analysis in routine and consultation practice settings with development of an algorithmic approach. *Am J Surg Pathol* 2009;33:805–17.

51 Hancock B W, Nazir K, Everard J E. Persistent gestational trophoblastic neoplasia after partial hydatidiform mole incidence and outcome. *J Reprod Med* 2006;51:764–6.

52 Feltmate C M, Growdon W B, Wolfberg A J, Goldstein D P, Genest D R, Chinchilla ME, et al. Clinical characteristics of persistent gestational trophoblastic neoplasia after partial hydatidiform molar pregnancy. *J Reprod Med* 2006;51:902–6.

53 Seckl M J, Fisher R A, Salerno G, Rees H, Paradinas F J, Foskett M, et al. Choriocarcinoma and partial hydatidiform moles. *Lancet* 2000;356:36–9.

54 Medeiros F, Callahan MJ, Elvin J A, Dorfman D M, Berkowitz R S, Quade B J. Intraplacental choriocarcinoma arising in a second trimester placenta with partial hydatidiform mole. *Int J Gynecol Pathol* 2008;27:247–51.

55 Garavaglia E, Gentile C, Cavoretto P, Spagnolo D, Valsecchi L, Mangili G. Ultrasound imaging after evacuation as an adjunct to beta-hCG monitoring in posthydatidiform molar gestational trophoblastic neoplasia. *Am J Obstet Gynecol* 2009;200:417.e1–5.

56 Lurain J R. Gestational trophoblastic disease I: epidemiology, pathology, clinical presentation and diagnosis of gestational trophoblastic disease, and management of hydatidiform mole. *Am J Obstet Gynecol* 2010;203:531–9.

57 Seckl M J, Sebire N J, Berkowitz R S. Gestational trophoblastic disease. *Lancet* 2010;376:717–29.

8 Drugs in early pregnancy

Neelam Potdar and Janine Elson

Introduction

Although most women are screened in the community and referred to high-risk consultant-led antenatal clinics if required, clinicians are faced with early pregnancy drug-exposure dilemmas when managing acute gynaecology emergencies. This chapter provides evidence-based knowledge regarding drug exposure in early pregnancy and help in improving the care of women in the emergency gynaecology setting (Box 8.1).

Pregnant women on average take between one and four medications during pregnancy, not including vitamins or minerals. About 80% of women use some form of medication during the first trimester of pregnancy.[1] Nearly 70% of these are over-the-counter medications and 30% are prescriptions.

Before prescribing medicines or over-the-counter drugs to pregnant women, it is important to understand the physiological changes during pregnancy that have a marked impact on the pharmacokinetics and placental transfer of drugs. Increased cardiovascular output and expansion of plasma volume reduce drug concentrations and the drug-binding capacity of the circulating proteins. Other changes include increased renal and endocrine function, reduced lung capacity and gastrointestinal motility and changes in liver metabolism. Finally, as the placenta is primarily a lipid barrier, many of the administered drugs cross the placenta by passive diffusion and reach the fetus. Low-molecular-weight, lipid-soluble, non-ionised drugs cross the placenta more readily. The effects of drug exposure during early pregnancy depend on the developmental stage of the embryo or fetus. There are three main stages in the development of the conceptus:[2]

- Predifferentiation or pre-embryonic stage (from conception until 17 days postconception). During this phase the cells divide rapidly

BOX 8.1 **Key clinical presentations related to drug exposure in early pregnancy**

- Pregnant women diagnosed de novo in early pregnancy who require treatment

- Pregnant women with a known disorder who are not on current medication and require treatment

- Pregnant women with a known disorder who are on medications started before pregnancy

- Pregnant women on medications taken for short-term conditions (contraception, methotrexate, antibiotics, etc.) and who have an unplanned pregnancy

TABLE 8.1 **US Food and Drug Administration classified drug use in pregnancy and risk categories**[4]

Class of drug	Recommendations
A	Controlled studies in women have failed to demonstrate risk to the fetus. Possibility of fetal risk appears remote.
B	Animal studies have not demonstrated fetal risk. There are no controlled studies in pregnant women, or animal studies have shown an adverse effect not confirmed in women.
C	Animal studies have demonstrated adverse effects on the fetus, and there are no controlled studies in pregnant women.
D	Studies have demonstrated evidence of human fetal risk. The use of this drug may be acceptable in life-threatening situations in the absence of safer drugs.
X	Studies have demonstrated fetal abnormalities. Risk from drug use clearly outweighs any possible benefit. Absolute contraindication in pregnancy.

and remain totipotent. The adverse effects of the drugs may damage a large number of cells and lead to miscarriage or, if the damage is to a small population of cells, those cells are replaced without any long-lasting damaging effect.

- Embryonic stage (from the 3rd to the 8th week postconception). During this stage the cells differentiate to form definitive organ systems. Drug insults cause lasting damage to the organs (congenital malformations); additionally, each organ system has a window of maximum susceptibility when the teratogenic insults are likely to be severe.

- Fetal stage (from the 9th week postconception until term). During this phase fetal tissues undergo growth and maturation. Adverse drug effects inhibit growth and can cause functional damage.

In principle, clinically indicated drugs should not be withheld from pregnant women if the expected benefit to the mother is considered to be greater than the risk to the fetus. On the other hand, unless absolutely necessary, drugs should be avoided in the first trimester. Drugs that have been used extensively during pregnancy and have proved to be safe should be prescribed in preference to new or untried medications. Lastly, the smallest effective dosage should be used.[3]

In the USA, the Food and Drug Administration has categorised drug use in pregnancy and the potential risk in five classes[4] (Table 8.1). However, these

TABLE 8.2 **Drugs with known teratogenic effects**

Drug	Teratogenic effect
Thalidomide	Phocomelia (absence of long bones from upper or lower limbs), external ear and heart defects [12]
Isotretinoin	Microtia, anotia, micrognathia, cleft palate, heart defects, eye anomalies, hydrocephalus, thymic agenesis, limb reduction defects [191,192]
Aminopterin	Short stature, craniosynostosis, hydrocephalus, hypertelorism, micrognathia, cleft palate [193]
Phenytoin	Craniofacial abnormalities, hypoplasia of distal phalanges and nails, growth deficiency, mental deficiency [83]
Warfarin	Nasal hypoplasia, stippled bone epiphyses, malformed vertebral bodies, microcephaly, ophthalmic anomalies [194,195]
Diethylstilbestrol	Females: vaginal adenosis, T-shaped uterus, uterine hypoplasia, incompetent cervix, clear-cell adenocarcinoma of vagina or cervix [196] Males: epididymal cyst, hypoplastic testes, cryptorchidism [197]

are only guidelines and should not form the basis of all prescriptions. Many newer drugs have not been tested in clinical trials and therefore their recommendation is based on observational or anecdotal studies. With the use of certain drugs, no evidence for a detrimental effect on pregnancy outcome has been demonstrated; however, lack of evidence does not mean that these drugs are without risk, and in many cases the British National Formulary advises avoiding their use in pregnancy. It is therefore essential for healthcare professionals to provide the mother with the best evidence available to help her make an informed decision.

Teratogenesis is defined as a structural or functional dysgenesis of fetal organs.[5] The typical manifestations include congenital malformations, intrauterine growth restriction, carcinogenesis and fetal demise. The effects of intrauterine drug exposure may be visible at the time of birth or may manifest later in life. The period of highest sensitivity to teratogenic effects is early organogenesis (days 17–35 postconception) so it is vital to establish the accurate gestational age of the fetus to ascertain the potential risk. Some of the known teratogenic drugs are listed in Table 8.2.

Nutritional supplements

Folic acid

Neural tube defects are among the most common birth defects.[6] A 2009 systematic review of evidence supports that folic acid supplementation reduced the risk of neural tube defects.[7] In this review, the odds ratio for a reduction in the incidence of neural tube defects with preconceptional folic acid supplementation ranged from 0.11 to 0.65. A concern with preconceptional folic acid intake is masking of vitamin B_{12} deficiency. To investigate this an ecological study compared patients before and after folic acid supplementation and found no evidence of an increase in low vitamin B_{12} concentrations without anaemia.[8]

Vitamin A

High levels of vitamin A (isoretinoin) in pregnancy are teratogenic (Table 8.2). The current recommendations are to inform pregnant women that vitamin A supplementation (more than 700 micrograms/day or 2310 iu) might be teratogenic, so it should be avoided. As liver and liver products may also contain high levels of vitamin A, consumption of these products in pregnancy should also be avoided.[9]

Drugs used for common early pregnancy ailments

Antiemetics

Nausea and vomiting in pregnancy affects 50–80% of women.[10] Depending on the severity, symptomatic treatment may be required. Various pharmacological modalities have been used but very few randomised controlled trials have compared their efficacy or effects on fetal outcome.[11] The evidence regarding their safety stems from large observational studies, case series and expert opinion.

Thalidomide
This is a hypnotic–sedative drug that was marketed from 1957 to 1961 and then withdrawn because of the confirmed teratogenic effects (Table 8.2). It was used as an effective painkiller, tranquiliser and antiemetic. In utero exposure between 27 and 42 days postconception produced phocomelia.[12] Current advice is to use contraception at least 1 month before, during and for 1 month after treatment with thalidomide (oral contraceptive pills are not recommended because of an increased risk of thromboembolism).

Antihistamines (H₁ receptor antagonists)
These agents act by direct inhibition of histamine binding at the central and peripheral H_1 receptors, thereby reducing nausea and vomiting in pregnancy.

Promethazine and cyclizine, first-generation non-selective antihistamines, are widely used. A large meta-analysis including data from 200 000 women has confirmed their efficacy with no increased risk of teratogenicity.[13] Maternal adverse effects include drowsiness, dry mouth, dizziness and extrapyramidal symptoms such as acute dystonic reactions involving facial and skeletal muscle spasms or oculogyric crises. Cetirizine and loratadine, second-generation antihistamines, are less sedative but are not recommended in early pregnancy because of insufficient evidence regarding safety. A recent meta-analysis ($n = 2694$ boys born to women exposed to loratadine during pregnancy) concluded that there is no risk of hypospadias associated with loratadine use during pregnancy.[14]

Phenothiazines

These drugs are dopamine receptor antagonists of both central and peripheral D_2 receptors and are used as antipsychotics and antiemetics. Prochlorperazine is safe in pregnancy[15] and can be prescribed sublingually or in suppository form. Chlorpromazine has been reported to increase the incidence of cleft defects in mice but not in humans.[16] Other antipsychotics such as levomepromazine and haloperidol do not have enough data for their safety in pregnancy to be assessed. Maternal adverse effects with use of phenothiazines include akathisia, tardive dyskinesia, extrapyramidal symptoms and substantial weight gain. Neuroleptic malignant syndrome is rare but potentially fatal.

Centrally acting dopamine antagonists such as metoclopramide and domperidone do not have a greater than expected risk of teratogenicity,[17] but they can cause extrapyramidal adverse effects. Manufacturers' advice is to avoid use of domperidone in pregnancy.

Serotonin inhibitors

Ondansetron, a selective serotonin 5 hydroxytryptamine 3 (5-HT3) receptor antagonist, has a central chemoreceptor inhibitory effect as well as peripheral action on the small bowel and vagus nerve. It is effective in relieving post-operative and chemotherapy-related nausea and vomiting.[18] Siu et al.[19] have demonstrated placental transfer of ondansetron during the first trimester of pregnancy, but there is no reported increase in fetal malformations above the baseline.[19,20] Several reports suggest the effectiveness of ondansetron in the treatment of hyperemesis gravidarum,[21,22] while others have shown it to be as effective as promethazine.[23] In view of insufficient evidence to support its safety, current guidance is to avoid the use of ondansetron unless the potential benefit outweighs the risk.

Vitamin B₆ (pyridoxine)

Vitamin B_6 in combination with an antihistamine (doxylamine) was marketed in Canada as Bendectin® (Merrell Dow Pharmaceuticals, Kansas City, MI, USA), and as Debendox® in the UK, for treating nausea and vomiting in pregnancy. In 1983 it was withdrawn from the market after its use was linked to limb defects in babies. However, it was later confirmed that the evidence did not provide support for its teratogenicity.[24,25] Randomised controlled trials suggest that vitamin B_6 reduces nausea and vomiting[26,27] and is safe for use in early pregnancy.[17,28]

Corticosteroids

Traditionally, corticosteroids have been used for the treatment of intractable hyperemesis. Corticosteroids vary in their ability to cross the placenta: betamethasone and dexamethasone cross the placenta readily, whereas 88% of prednisone is metabolised in the placenta.[3] Early studies suggested the possibility of fetal cleft defects with the use of corticosteroids in pregnancy; however, the Committee on Safety of Medicines concluded that there is no convincing evidence of an increased incidence of congenital abnormalities such as cleft palate or lip with corticosteroid use.[3]

There are conflicting reports regarding the efficacy of corticosteroids in the treatment of nausea and vomiting in pregnancy. Some studies have shown no difference in effect compared with antihistamines,[29,30] whereas others have shown benefit with the use of pulsed corticosteroid therapy.[31]

Antacids and proton pump inhibitors

Approximately 22% of women suffer from heartburn in early pregnancy, which usually requires pharmacotherapy.[32] Antacids are effective as they neutralise and bind bile acids. Alginate preparations of antacids, such as Gaviscon® (Reckitt Benckiser, Slough, Berks, UK), inhibit gastric content regurgitation and are safe during pregnancy.[33]

H_2 receptor blockers such as ranitidine and cimetidine reduce acid secretion and volume and are effective and safe in early pregnancy.[34] In a cohort of 178 women, no association between cimetidine use and fetal malformations was shown,[35] although an antiandrogenic effect has been demonstrated in rats.[36] Current advice is to avoid the use of ranitidine and cimetidine unless essential. There are limited data on the safety of famotidine and nizatidine in pregnancy, so they should not be prescribed.

Proton pump inhibitors, such as omeprazole, suppress gastric acid secretion and are effective in reducing severe heartburn. A meta-analysis of five cohort studies reported no association between exposure to proton pump inhibitors and fetal malformations.[37,38] In dosages higher than those used in humans it has been associated with embryotoxicity in animals; therefore, the advice is for cautious use in pregnancy.[33]

Laxatives and antidiarrhoeals

Forty percent of women report symptoms of constipation at 14 weeks of gestation. Diet modifications with bran or wheat fibre supplementation are recommended options.[39] There is no evidence available for the effectiveness and safety of osmotic laxatives, such as lactulose, or softeners in pregnancy.[39] Long-term use of saline osmotic laxatives such as magnesium citrate and sodium phosphate should be avoided. For chronic constipation in pregnancy, polyethylene glycol is considered safe.

Antidiarrhoeals such as loperamide, diphenoxylate and bismuth-containing compounds should be avoided because of their risk of fetotoxicity.

Analgesics

Paracetamol
Paracetamol is widely used in pregnancy for analgesia and as an antipyretic. At normal therapeutic dosages, no teratogenic effects have been reported.[40] It can be taken safely throughout pregnancy.

Aspirin
In early pregnancy, low-dose aspirin is used as prophylaxis for severe pre-eclampsia, fetal growth restriction and prevention of pregnancy loss in women with thrombophilic antiphospholipid antibody syndrome. Evidence suggests that aspirin at low doses is safe for the fetus and at the recommended dosages is unlikely to increase the risk of congenital malformations.[41–44] Maternal adverse effects include upper gastrointestinal intolerability, worsening of asthma and Reye syndrome. Aspirin can exacerbate bleeding later in pregnancy.

Non-steroidal anti-inflammatory drugs
Ibuprofen, diclofenac and indomethacin belong to the non-steroidal anti-inflammatory class of drugs (NSAIDs). They are mainly prostaglandin synthesis inhibitors with action on the gut, kidneys and platelets. Animal studies have found no evidence of increased teratogenicity with the use of ketoprofen, ibuprofen and naproxen. Where possible, their use should be avoided in pregnancy as they are inhibitors of prostaglandin synthesis and long-term use can

cause haemostatic abnormalities and premature closure of the ductus arteriosus or persistent pulmonary artery hypertension in the newborn infant.[45]

Opioid analgesics

Some of the opioid analgesics, such as morphine, pethidine, fentanyl, hydromorphine and oxycodone, are considered safe for use in early pregnancy.[46] However, use of codeine and propoxyphene (an ingredient of co-proxamol) has been associated with fetal malformations.[46] Over the years, large exposures to codeine have not demonstrated teratogenic effects, and it can be prescribed in pregnancy.[3]

Anti-migraine drugs

Migraine attacks are most frequent during the first trimester of pregnancy.[47,48] Drugs used for the treatment of migraine include opioid analgesics, NSAIDs, ergot alkaloids, isometheptene and selective serotonin 5-HT1B/1D receptor agonists (triptans).

Paracetamol is the mainstay of treatment for a typical episode during early pregnancy. Ergot alkaloids (including methysergide) are associated with miscarriage and birth defects of intestinal atresia,[49] poor cerebral development and Möbius syndrome.[50,51] These drugs are contraindicated in pregnancy. Caffeine is used in combination with other drugs for the short-term treatment of migraine. Epidemiological evidence suggests that high dosages of caffeine (over 300 mg/day) can cause miscarriage; therefore, it should not be consumed beyond the recommended dose.[52,53] Isometheptene, a sympathomimetic agent with non-specific adrenoceptor agonist effects, is administered in combination with paracetamol and dichloralphenazone for the treatment of migraine. There are no reports of its teratogenicity, but it is less effective in pregnancy.[54]

Sumatriptan, a selective serotonin 5-HT1B/1D receptor agonist, is relatively hydrophilic and only 15% of the administered dose crosses the placenta.[55] Evidence regarding the efficacy and safety of sumatriptan comes from epidemiological and pharmacovigilance studies and pregnancy registries. None of the studies has suggested an increase in miscarriages or fetal malformations.[56] Sumatriptan can be used in early pregnancy with caution, whereas all other 5-HT receptor agonists should be avoided owing to the lack of safety information.

Propranolol is prescribed for the prophylactic treatment of migraine (see the section on antihypertensives below). In non-pregnant women, prophylactic medication provides a 50% reduction in the number of migraine attacks but, in pregnancy, anti-migraine drugs should be prescribed only when absolutely indicated.

Vaccines

Immunisation is generally avoided in pregnancy. Vaccines made with live virus (rubella and varicella) are contraindicated in pregnancy and conception should be avoided in the month following vaccination. Killed vaccines (hepatitis A and B, plague, rabies, tetanus, diphtheria and typhoid) can be given to pregnant women if there is a substantial risk of infection.

Swine flu (H1N1) was first associated with pigs but has been transmitted to humans and spread as a pandemic in 2009. Pregnant women are particularly vulnerable to H1N1 influenza and are more likely to be admitted to hospital. In the acute phase, women can use paracetamol for symptomatic relief. As a preventative measure, the Department of Health strongly recommends that pregnant women have the vaccine to protect both mother and baby.[57] Correct information about the advantages and safety of vaccination should be available to help women make informed choices.

Two types of vaccine are available, Pandemrix™ (GlaxoSmithKline, Brentford, Middlesex, UK) and Celvapan (Baxter, Deerfield, IL, USA). Pandemrix has an active antigen derived from H1N1 and contains an immunological adjuvant, AS03, whereas Celvapan contains H1N1 viruses that have been inactivated. Pandemrix is given as a single dose and Celvapan is given in two doses at least 3 weeks apart. The Joint Committee on Vaccinations and Immunisation recommends Pandemrix for pregnant women as the single-dose schedule gives excellent and rapid protection against the virus. According to the expert scientific advice, thiomersal, contained in Pandemrix, does not present a risk to pregnant women or their babies.[57]

Antifungals

Vaginal candidiasis caused by *Candida albicans* is a frequent infection in pregnancy. A week-long course of topical imidazoles (clotrimazole and econazole) is an effective treatment.[39] Exposure to single or short doses of oral fluconazole during the first trimester is not associated with congenital malformations.[58] However, fetal malformations have been reported with long-term use of fluconazole in the first trimester.[59] As the effectiveness and safety of oral treatments for candidiasis in pregnancy are uncertain, they should not be prescribed.

Antibiotics

Chlamydia

The drugs of choice for the treatment of *Chlamydia trachomatis* are tetracyclines, but they are contraindicated in pregnancy because of their association with teeth and bone abnormalities. Erythromycin has been recommended as the first-line treatment, but evidence from a 2009 Cochrane review demonstrated that amoxicillin is as effective as erythromycin in achieving cure (OR 0.54, 95% CI 0.28–1.02).[60] Additionally, amoxicillin is better tolerated than erythromycin. Clindamycin and azithromycin should be considered if use of the above two drugs is contraindicated.

Bacterial vaginosis and trichomonal vaginitis

Once a diagnosis of bacterial vaginosis or trichomonal vaginitis is confirmed in pregnancy, treatment should be initiated. Metronidazole is the treatment of choice and, although it carries a theoretical risk of abnormalities, no problems have been reported from observational data.

Gonorrhoea

Gonorrhoea should be treated with penicillin or a third-generation cephalosporin such as cefotaxime or ceftriaxone.

Pelvic inflammatory disease

Pelvic inflammatory disease can be diagnosed in pregnancy, especially with the opportunistic screening performed during assessment of early pregnancy problems. The treatment regimen for non-pregnant women includes tetracyclines together with a cephalosporin and metronidazole. In pregnancy an acceptable alternative would be a third-generation cephalosporin with erythromycin and metronidazole.[61]

In cases of severe sepsis, the maternal benefit from treatment outweighs any fetal risk; therefore, the most appropriate antibiotic combination should be prescribed. In most cases an intravenous third-generation cephalosporin and metronidazole along with gentamicin are used. Careful monitoring of serum gentamicin concentrations is required to avoid maternal and fetal toxicity.

Quinolones such as ciprofloxacin, ofloxacin, levofloxacin and norfloxacin are associated with cartilage and joint defects in animal studies. In humans, a recent meta-analysis ($n = 984$) found no increase in the risk of major congenital malformations and other adverse pregnancy outcomes after first-trimester exposure to quinolones.[62] However, their use should be avoided as safer alternatives are available.[3]

Urinary tract infections

Urinary tract infections are common in pregnancy and if left untreated can escalate to acute pyelonephritis and other ascending infections. The most common organisms are Gram-positive and Gram-negative bacteria, especially *Escherichia coli*. The combination of trimethoprim–sulfonamide (TMP-SMX) is the first line of treatment in non-pregnant women. Both antibiotics are folic acid antagonists and inhibit nucleic acid synthesis in bacterial cells. Although the action of TMP-SMX is specific to bacteria, studies have reported an increased association of neural tube defects and cardiac defects when used in early pregnancy.[63,64] TMP-SMX should be avoided in the first trimester and substituted with other antibiotics, such as penicillins, cephalosporins, nitrofurantoin and macrolides.[65] In extreme clinical situations, if TMP-SMX is required in the first trimester, high-dose folic acid should be supplemented.

Tuberculosis

Isoniazid use is considered safe in pregnancy, but teratogenicity is suspected with rifampin and ethambutol. The recommendations are to prescribe first-line antituberculosis treatment as used in non-pregnant women.[66] Streptomycin is contraindicated in pregnancy because of ototoxicity in the fetus.[67] Ethionamide and prothionamide are prescribed only if their use is essential for the success of treatment.

Malaria

In animal studies, chloroquine compounds have been shown to cross the placenta and accumulate in the fetal uveal tract.[68] As their teratogenic effects are dose-related, they are considered safe when used weekly at prophylactic doses.[69] Pregnant women travelling to endemic areas should commence chloroquine 1 week before travelling and continue for 1 month after leaving the area. Chloroquine can be combined with daily proguanil, which is also considered safe in pregnancy. In chloroquine-resistant infections, mefloquine or sulphone/diaminopyrimidine with folic acid can be used with caution. If taken in the first trimester of pregnancy, proper counselling should be provided, and this should not be a reason for termination.[70] Although quinine is considered teratogenic in high doses, it can be used for treatment in pregnancy as the benefit outweighs the associated risks.

Toxoplasmosis

Infection in the first trimester is uncommon but severe. Maternal infection can be treated with spiramycin for 3 weeks. If fetal infection is suspected, pyrimethamine and sulfadiazine are added for 3 weeks with folic acid supplementation.

TABLE 8.3 **Commonly administered antiretroviral drugs**

Class	Drugs	Adverse effects
Nucleoside and nucleotide reverse transcriptase inhibitors	Zidovudine, didanosine, stavudine, lamivudine, abacavir, tenofovir, adefovir	Generally well tolerated. May cause mitochondrial dysfunction leading to lactic acidosis and hepatic toxicity. This is highest with zalcitabine, followed by didanosine, stavudine, lamivudine, zidovudine and abacavir.[198]
Non-nucleoside reverse transcriptase inhibitors	Efavirenz, nevirapine, delavirdine	Cutaneous and hepatic toxicity. A few hepatitis-related deaths with use for nausea and vomiting of pregnancy.[199]
Protease inhibitors	Saquinavir, ritonavir, nelfinavir, indinavir	Hyperglycaemia, new-onset diabetes, exacerbation of existing diabetes mellitus and diabetic ketoacidosis.[200,201]

Syphilis

Treatment in early pregnancy does not differ from most of the standard treatment regimens with penicillin.

HIV infection

The prevalence of HIV infection among pregnant women in the UK has increased in the first decade of the 21st century. A growing proportion of infected women are already diagnosed before they conceive.[71] More than 20 antiretroviral drugs are licensed for the specific treatment of HIV-1 infection in the UK and, of these, zidovudine is specifically indicated in pregnancy. The efficacy of zidovudine in reducing mother-to-child transmission of HIV-1 has been demonstrated in several large randomised controlled studies[72–74] and supported by epidemiological surveys.[75,76]

Antiretroviral drugs are broadly classified by the phase of the retrovirus life-cycle that the drug inhibits (Table 8.3). These can be administered as monotherapy or as a combination of drugs known as highly active antiretroviral therapy. Box 8.2 outlines the guidelines for prescribing antiretrovirals in pregnancy.

The Antiretroviral Pregnancy Registry contains a summary of relevant mutagenesis, carcinogenesis and teratogenesis data for each licensed antiretroviral agent (www.apregistry.com). Apart from didanosine and efavirenz no other compounds have given rise to concern. With didanosine the number of first-trimester exposures is relatively low, but the 95% CIs (3.3–9.4%) remain above the expected rate of 'early' congenital malformations (2.4%). The observed incidence of 5.8% also exceeds that observed with initiation of therapy in the second or third trimester (1%).[71] No specific pattern of congenital malformations has been observed. The concerns relating to efavirenz date to preclinical studies in macaques. First-trimester efavirenz exposure was associated with spinal cord and central nervous system malformations.[71] Until more robust data are available it is advisable to avoid efavirenz preconceptionally. After stopping the drug it can take up to 3 weeks for efavirenz to clear from the plasma. It is not known whether the first 6 weeks post-conception is the key period during which efavirenz affects central nervous system development. It is not known whether discontinuing efavirenz after confirmation of pregnancy will reduce the risk of spina bifida.

> **BOX 8.2 British HIV Association guidelines for HIV treatment in pregnancy**[71]
>
> ○ Asymptomatic women who do not require antiretroviral treatment for their own health may be treated with short-duration highly active antiretroviral therapy (HAART) commencing in the second trimester.
>
> ○ Women who require HAART for their own health should commence treatment early, although it can be deferred until after the first trimester.
>
> ○ If a mother conceives on HAART, has an undetectable viral load and is tolerating the combination well, she should be encouraged to continue this regimen, even if it contains efavirenz (www.apregistry.com).[202]

System-specific drugs used in early pregnancy

Anti-epileptics

Anti-epileptics are used to treat epilepsy, headaches and mood disorders in women of reproductive age. Often the treatment needs to be continued in pregnancy to avoid serious complications of seizures and trauma. Most anti-epileptics are known to increase the risk of major congenital malformations (4–7%),[77] specific congenital syndromes, minor anomalies and developmental cognitive and behavioural disorders in childhood.[78] The risks are highest in women receiving polypharmacy,[79] valproate[80] and phenobarbital.[81] However, research with the newer anti-epileptics suggests equivalent, if not safer, profiles compared with the older drugs.

The most common major malformations with antiepileptics include cardiac defects, urogenital malformations, craniofacial defects and skeletal abnormalities.[82] Fetal anticonvulsant syndrome has been reported with the use of valproate, phenytoin,[83] carbamazepine[84] and phenobarbital.[85] The syndromes are generally similar with all antiepileptics and include a low or broad nasal bridge, epicanthic folds, hypertelorism, low hairline, hypoplasia of the distal phalanges and cognitive developmental anomalies.[86]

Valproate

Evidence for the greater teratogenic potential of valproate came from case series of spina bifida in children exposed to valproate in utero in the early 1980s.[87] Since then, several publications have confirmed these findings.[88,89] A prospective study – the Neurodevelopmental Effects of Antiepileptic Drugs (NEAD) – has confirmed the increased risk of major malformations with valproate and its dose-dependent effect (20.3% with valproate versus 10.7% with phenytoin, 8.2% with carbamazepine and 1% with lamotrigine).[80] Based on the evidence, recommendations are not to use valproate as a first-line medication in women of childbearing years; if used, the dose should be limited.

Phenobarbitone

Phenobarbitone is one of the oldest anti-epileptics in use. The risk of major congenital malformations is higher with the use of phenobarbitone compared with the general population (11%) and a possible dose–response relationship exists with doses greater than 60 mg/day.[90] Subsequent studies have confirmed these findings.[85]

Phenytoin

The hydantoin syndrome in fetuses exposed to phenytoin is well documented.[83] The risk of malformations is two to three times greater than that seen in the general population,[80] hence its use in pregnancy is contraindicated.

Carbamazepine

The risks associated with carbamazepine are similar to those of phenytoin apart from the increased risk of neural tube defects.[91] In a systematic review of women exposed to oxocarbazepine, there was no evidence of an increased risk of major malformations with monotherapy (2.4%) versus its use in polytherapy (6.6%).[92]

Benzodiazepines

The evidence regarding the teratogenicity of benzodiazepines is inconclusive. A large meta-analysis of 12 cohort studies of benzodiazepine exposure in utero showed no increase in the risk of major abnormalities or cleft lip (OR 0.9, 95% CI 0.61–1.35).[93] However, a meta-analysis of case–control studies showed a risk increment (OR 3.01, 95% CI 1.32–6.84).[93]

Lamotrigine

Lamotrigine is one of the newer anti-epileptics, having been used since the 1990s. The NEAD study demonstrated that lamotrigine exposure in pregnancy

compared favourably to other anti-epileptics, with a 1% risk of major malformations, and there was no increased risk compared with women not taking
anti-epileptics. Although an early report from the International Lamotrigine
Pregnancy Registry suggested a dose–response effect of lamotrigine, a more
recent report from the same registry concluded that there was no evidence
of an increased risk of major malformations with lamotrigine exposure (2.9%
over 800 exposures).[94]

Other anti-epileptics and polypharmacy

Data on exposure to levetiracetam, gabapentin, topiramate and vigabatrin during pregnancy are small and variable; therefore, the use of these drugs in pregnancy is not recommended. There is sufficient evidence regarding an increased
risk of teratogenesis with polypharmacy compared with monotherapy.[79]

Although the relative risks of major malformations are increased for
women taking anti-epileptics, the absolute risks are low. Pregnant women
should be prescribed the minimal effective dosage, avoiding polypharmacy
where possible. Serum concentrations of the drugs should be followed in
pregnancy to avoid toxicity and to check for compliance and for dose adjust-
ment. While there is evidence to suggest that women on anti-epileptics and
low levels of folate are at risk of major malformations and neural tube defects,
folate supplementation has not been shown to decrease the risk, particularly
for valproate.[95] Nevertheless, high-dose folate (5 mg/day) is recommended
for women taking enzyme-inducing anti-epileptics (carbamazepine, phenytoin and phenobarbital) or valproate. Women trying for a pregnancy who are
taking these drugs should be referred to specialists for counselling and, once
pregnant, should be offered screening for neural tube defects in early pregnancy by serum alphafetoprotein and ultrasonography.

Antihypertensives

Approximately 1% of hypertensive disorders present as pre-existing or chronic
hypertension in pregnancy.[96] In early pregnancy, blood pressure falls physiologically due to general relaxation of muscles within the blood vessels,[97]
obviating the need to continue antihypertensive medication. However, persistently raised blood pressure in early pregnancy requires treatment to prevent
maternal vascular damage and to avoid the risk of miscarriage and placental
insufficiency. The aim of treatment is to bring about a smooth reduction in
blood pressure that is safe for both the mother and the fetus. Depending on
the severity of hypertension, a wide variety of drugs is advocated, each with
potential adverse effects.

Centrally acting antihypertensives

Methyldopa is a centrally acting first-line drug for the treatment of hypertension and is considered the safest antihypertensive in pregnancy.[98] It crosses the placenta freely and reaches cord blood in similar concentrations to those seen in the mother.[99] It has been used for decades and there is evidence regarding its safety from follow-up studies.[100] Preconceptionally, methyldopa is considered as a drug of choice for treating hypertension, unless contraindicated. Maternal adverse effects include depression, drowsiness, fluid retention, postural hypotension and, rarely, autoimmune haemolytic anaemia and systemic lupus erythematosus-like syndrome. Women suffering from prenatal depression should be prescribed alternative medication.

Clonidine is a centrally acting alpha agonist but has the disadvantage of causing hypertensive crises with sudden withdrawal.[101]

Beta-blockers

Beta-blockers are beta receptor antagonists that inhibit epinephrine-mediated sympathetic actions in various organs, including the heart and vascular smooth muscle. Their antihypertensive action involves a reduction of cardiac output, renin release and sympathetic activity. Some of the drugs in this group are atenolol, propranolol, metoprolol and acebutolol. In pregnancy, beta-blockers commonly cross the placenta and may cause lowering of the fetal heart rate. If commenced in early pregnancy they may cause fetal growth restriction [102,103] and low birth weight, although the reported effects vary.[104,105]

Labetalol has a mixed beta and alpha-1 adrenergic receptor antagonistic activity, which provides an additional arteriolar vasodilating effect. It is safe for use in pregnancy,[106,107] but can cause maternal fatigue and orthostatic hypotension and can worsen bronchial asthma.[108]

Calcium channel blockers

Calcium channel blockers inhibit calcium ion influx in the vascular smooth muscle, resulting in arterial vasodilation. Nifedipine, nicardipine, nimodipine and isradipine have all been used in pregnancy. Their use in early pregnancy is not associated with an increased risk of fetal malformation.[109] Maternal adverse effects include headache and sudden hypotension; therefore, these drugs should be used carefully. Verapamil, another calcium channel blocker, has a predominant negative chronotropic action and is used for the treatment of paroxysmal supraventricular tachycardia. As there is limited information regarding fetal safety, verapamil should be substituted with other drugs.

Angiotensin-converting enzyme inhibitors

Angiotensin-converting enzyme inhibitors comprise enalapril, captopril and lisinopril. These drugs are renoprotective and are used as first-line medications in diabetes with microalbuminuria or nephropathy. They are contraindicated in pregnancy as there is evidence of oligohydramnios, fetal anuria, congenital renal dysgenesis [110] and stillbirths with their use.[111,112] Interestingly, if use is limited to the first trimester, these drugs do not present the risk of teratogenicity.[113–115] However, women who are planning to become pregnant should be prescribed alternative drugs.

Angiotensin 2 receptor antagonists

There are insufficient data regarding the safety of this class of antihypertensives (valsartan and losartan) in pregnancy and therefore they should not be prescribed.

Diuretics

In the general population diuretics are the first-line antihypertensives. They are not used in pregnancy because of the risk of reduction in the intravascular blood volume and effect on the uteroplacental blood flow.[116] No direct adverse fetal effects have been reported.[117] These drugs are reserved for pregnant women with specific renal or cardiac problems.[118]

Anti-psychotics

Treatment with anti-psychotics during pregnancy requires assessment of the clinical effectiveness of the drug and the risk of toxicity to the mother and fetus.[119] A decision to withhold medication can result in exacerbation of symptoms and increased risk of self-harm. The risk of harm to the offspring associated with in utero exposure to these drugs is unknown.[120] Current guidelines for the use of anti-psychotics are based on evidence from observational data rather than randomised controlled trials.

Antidepressants

Tricyclic antidepressants are the oldest psychoactive drugs. Discovered in the early 1950s, they are used for the treatment of major depression, dysthymia, bipolar and other anxiety and eating disorders. They act as serotonin–norepinehrine reuptake inhibitors, resulting in elevation of the extracellular concentrations of these neurotransmitters. Many drugs are included in this class, but medications commonly used in pregnancy include amitriptyline and imipramine. Teratogenicity has been shown in animals; however, in observational human studies their safety has been confirmed, even with exposure in the first trimester.[121] They are the preferred choice of antidepressants in pregnancy as they have been used over a long period of time and there are data to suggest safety in humans. Maternal adverse effects include dry mouth, blurred vision, constipation, urinary retention, drowsiness, akathisia, sexual dysfunction and changes in weight and appetite.

Selective serotonin reuptake inhibitors

Selective serotonin reuptake inhibitors are the newer class of antidepressants, which increase the extracellular level of serotonin by inhibiting its reuptake and increasing serotonin binding at the postsynaptic receptor. Drugs in this class include citalopram, fluoxetine, paroxetine, sertraline, venlafaxine and mirtazapine. It takes 6–8 weeks for the full onset of action of these drugs. The general adverse effects include nausea, anhedonia, apathy, drowsiness and urinary retention and these are present mostly for the first 1–4 weeks of use.

Fluoxetine has been prescribed for more than a decade. Observational data are available regarding its efficacy and safety in pregnancy.[121] Animal data in the past suggested an increased risk of craniofacial abnormalities with high doses, but most human studies have shown it to be safe.[122,123]

There are conflicting reports regarding the safety of paroxetine in pregnancy. A meta-analysis found first-trimester paroxetine exposure to be associated with a significantly increased risk of fetal cardiac malformation,[124] while another study did not find evidence of increased risk of congenital malformations.[125] The results of a systematic review have refuted the findings of the earlier meta-analysis and concluded that the positive association may be due to publication bias.[126]

Safety data on the newer antidepressants such as venlafaxine are limited; therefore, they should be substituted or prescribed only if the maternal benefit outweighs the risks.

Lithium

Lithium is used for the treatment of bipolar mood disorder. Concerns regarding its teratogenicity were raised in the late 1960s. A meta-analysis found an increased relative risk of Ebstein's anomaly (1/1000–2000 compared with 1/20 000 in the general population) following first-trimester exposure to lithium, although the absolute risk remains very small.[127] Other reported malformations include obstructed hydrocephalus, ear atresia, club feet, maxillary hypoplasia and meningomyelocele. Women who are on lithium preconceptionally should taper their dose gradually on confirmation of pregnancy as there is a risk of rebound psychosis with sudden withdrawal.[128] Once lithium is stopped and the mood disorder is under control, supportive psychological methods should be offered. If the mood disorder is severe, the woman may require hospitalisation, initiation of lithium or other psychotropic medication and, sometimes, elctroconvulsive therapy. If lithium needs to be continued for maternal benefit, fetal echocardiography should be organised at 18–22 weeks of gestation.

Neuroleptics

Neuroleptics are used for the treatment of schizophrenia and include chlorpro-mazine, haloperidol and trifluoperazine. Conflicting evidence exists regarding their safety in early pregnancy.[129] Relative risks for congenital abnormalities have been shown to be high with neuroleptics. No specific organ defects have been identified.[130] Atypical neuroleptics such as clozapine, risperidone, quetiapine and olanzapine are best avoided because of the limited data on their safety in pregnancy. Atypical neuroleptic agents taken preconceptionally should be changed to conventional high-dose alternatives as soon as pregnancy is confirmed. In refractory cases continuation of the atypical neuroleptics may be required if the benefits outweigh the associated risks.

Treatment of endocrine disorders

Hypothyroidism

Most women with hypothyroidism are diagnosed before pregnancy and are on thyroid hormone replacement with levothyroxine. The fetus is dependent on maternal thyroxine until 10–12 weeks of gestation, when it starts secreting thyroid hormones from its own thyroid gland.[131] Thyroxine should be continued at the same dosage during pregnancy,[132] with assessment of thyroid function once in each trimester.

Hyperthyroidism (thyrotoxicosis)

Hyperthyroidism occurs in 1–2/1000 pregnant women. In 80–85% of cases it is due to thyrotoxicosis.[133] Thyrotoxicosis secondary to Graves' disease worsens during the first trimester of pregnancy and improves as pregnancy progresses. The aim of treatment is to maintain maternal free thyroxine in the upper normal range using the lowest possible dosage of the anti-thyroid drug to avoid fetal hypothyroidism. Propylthiouracil, carbimazole and methimazole are the antithyroid drugs used for treatment. Radioactive iodine is contraindicated as it crosses the placenta and is taken up by the fetal thyroid gland. In cases of treatment failure or adverse drug effects, thyroidectomy is indicated, usually in the second trimester.

TABLE 8.4 **Oral hypoglycaemic agents and their safety in pregnancy**

Class	Drugs	Placental transfer and safety[203]
Sulphonylureas	Chlorpropamide, glibenclamide, glimepiride, glipizide, tolbutamide	Chlorpropamide and tolbutamide: present a risk to the fetus (neonatal hypoglycaemia) if taken in third trimester.
		Glibenclamide: potentially safe.
		Glimerpiride: no studies.
		Glipizide: no evidence of increased risk of malformations.
Biguanides	Metformin	Crosses placenta.
		Systematic reviews do not show an increased risk of teratogenicity.
Alpha-glucosidase inhibitors	Acarbose	Observational studies show some evidence of congenital malformation.
Thiazolidinediones	Pioglitazone, rosiglitazone	No studies. May cause postimplantation losses.
Insulin-release stimulators	Nateglinide, repaglinide	One case report suggests low risk of developmental toxicity.

Propylthiouracil is a highly protein-bound drug with limited transplacental passage compared with other antithyroid drugs. It is considered safe in pregnancy, with no teratogenic effects. Methimazole, an active compound of carbimazole, has been associated with teratogenic effects in some epidemiological studies.[134,135] Congenital abnormalities are characterised by aplasia cutis, facial abnormalities, oesophageal atresia and developmental delay.[136] However, other studies have not found this association in infants exposed to methimazole in utero.[137,138] In women who cannot tolerate propylthiouracil, methimazole has been used as an alternative.

Diabetes and hypoglycaemic drugs

Diabetes affects 2–5% of pregnancies and of these approximately 87.5% is due to gestational diabetes, 7.5% to type I diabetes and the remaining 5% to type II diabetes.[139]

ORAL HYPOGLYCAEMIC AGENTS

Oral hypoglycaemic agents are used for the treatment of type II diabetes (Table 8.4). In a meta-analysis of first-trimester exposure to oral hypoglycaemic agents and occurrence of subsequent major congenital abnormalities, there was no significant difference between exposed and unexposed women (10 studies, OR 1.05, 95% CI 0.65–1.70).[140] A systematic review on the use of metformin in the first trimester reported no increase in the incidence of major malformations.[141] Furthermore, use of metformin during pregnancy in women with polycystic ovary syndrome is associated with a reduction in the miscarriage rate, maternal weight, fasting serum insulin levels and incidence of gestational diabetes. Evidence from retrospective data also suggests the safety of metformin and glibenclamide in pregnancy.[142]

INSULIN

Insulin is recommended as the drug of choice for pregnant women with diabetes. Insulin analogues are synthetic insulins that are either fast-acting preprandial insulin or long-acting basal insulin. The insulin analogues currently licensed in the UK are the fast-acting lispro, aspart and glulisine and the long-acting detemir and glargine. Some studies have shown insulin aspart to be effective in pregnancy without increasing the risk of hypoglycaemia and have shown insulin lispro to be non-teratogenic. There is a lack of evidence regarding the use of glulisine, glargine or detemir in pregnancy.

The National Institute for Health and Clinical Excellence has provided guidelines for the treatment of diabetes in pregnancy, which are summarised in Box 8.3.

BOX 8.3 **National Institute for Health and Clinical Excellence guidelines for use of hypoglycaemic drugs in pregnancy**[203]

○ Pregnant women with diabetes may be advised to use metformin as an adjunct or alternative to insulin when the likely benefits from improved glycaemic control outweigh the potential for harm.

○ All other oral hypoglycaemic agents should be discontinued and substituted with insulin.

○ Isophane insulin (neutral protamine Hagedorn or NPH insulin) remains the first-choice long-acting insulin during pregnancy as there is insufficient evidence for long-acting insulin analogues.

○ Rapid-acting insulin analogues (aspart and lispro) have advantages over soluble human insulin during pregnancy and their use should be considered.

○ Women with insulin-treated diabetes should be advised of the risks of hypoglycaemia and hypoglycaemia unawareness in pregnancy, particularly in the first trimester.

MEDICATIONS USED FOR COMPLICATIONS OF DIABETES

Angiotensin-converting enzyme inhibitors and angiotensin 2 receptor antagonists should be discontinued and alternative antihypertensives substituted. Statins should be discontinued before pregnancy or as soon as pregnancy is confirmed.

Hyperprolactinaemia

Dopaminergic agents such as bromocriptine and cabergoline are used for the management of pathological hyperprolactinaemia. Bromocriptine crosses the placenta, but there are no reported adverse fetal effects from its use in pregnancy.[143,144] Maternal complications of myocardial infarction and stroke have been reported; therefore, bromocriptine use should be avoided in women with hypertension. Limited experience is available for use of cabergoline in pregnancy.

Cushing syndrome

Metyrapone, trilostane and aminoglutethimide are the drugs used for the treatment of Cushing syndrome as they suppress the release of corticotrophin-releasing hormone. There is evidence for the safety of metyrapone use in the first trimester.[145] Trilostane is associated with an increased risk of miscarriage and should be avoided in pregnancy.[146] Similarly, aminoglutethimide should be avoided in pregnancy as animal studies have shown teratogenic effects and pseudohermaphroditism is reported in female infants exposed to the drug in utero.

Anticoagulants

Heparin

Unfractionated heparin is a mucopolysaccharide with a high molecular weight (4000–40 000). It is used for thromboprophylaxis because of its antithrombotic and antiplatelet activity. Once fractionated, heparin is converted to low-molecular-weight heparins, which have greater anti-Xa activity and minimal antiplatelet effect. Neither form of heparin crosses the placenta[147] and both forms are safe for the fetus. Heparin is administered subcutaneously and can cause pain and slight bruising at the injection sites. Other uncommon maternal risks include bleeding, heparin-induced thrombocytopenia and heparin-induced osteopenia with fractures.

Warfarin

Warfarin is a coumarin derivative with vitamin K antagonistic activity that is used for long-term thromboprophylaxis. It crosses the placenta freely and carries a known risk of teratogenicity. The most common syndrome is chondrodysplasia punctata, with abnormal bone and cartilage formation.[148] Other defects include asplenia and diaphragmatic hernia. In high doses it can cause fetal intracerebral bleed, leading to optic atrophy, microcephaly and restricted neurological development.[149] Furthermore, there is evidence that warfarin use is associated with an increased risk of miscarriage.[150] Ideally, warfarin should be avoided in pregnancy. In women with artificial heart valves warfarin is the anticoagulant of choice, and its use at the dosage needed to maintain an international normalised ratio of 3 may reduce the risk of teratogenicity and miscarriage[151] without compromising the antithrombotic effect.[152] In some studies, warfarin has been substituted with heparin (subcutaneous or infu-

TABLE 8.5 **Anti-rheumatic drugs used for treatment of rheumatic disorders**

Drugs	Disorders
NSAIDs	Osteoarthritis, inflammatory arthritis
Antimalarials	SLE, RA
Sulfasalazine	RA, ankylosing spondylitis
Penicillamine	Severe RA, psoriatic arthritis
Corticosteroids	SLE, RA
Gold salts	Severe RA, psoriatic arthritis
Cytotoxic drugs	SLE, unremitting RA

NSAIDs = non-steroidal anti-inflammatory drugs | RA = rheumatic arthritis | SLE = systemic lupus erythmatosus.

sion) until the end of 12 weeks of gestation and then recommenced until the end of pregnancy.[151,153] Appropriate counselling regarding warfarin use is crucial in pregnant women with artificial heart valves.

Treatment of rheumatic disorders

Rheumatic disorders are more common in women than in men, with the peak prevalence of certain disorders occurring in the reproductive years. Different classes of drugs are used depending on the type and severity of the disease (Table 8.5). Adequate control of the disease in pregnancy is vital. Pregnancy may cause remission of some disorders, whereas others require more aggressive treatment.

NSAIDS
Refer to the section on analgesics for information on the use of NSAIDs in pregnancy (page 91).

Sulfasalazine
Sulfasalazine is increasingly being used as a second-line drug in pregnant women with rheumatoid arthritis and inflammatory bowel disease. It crosses the placenta[154] and there is evidence regarding its safety when used in early pregnancy.[155,156] Although there are few case reports of congenital malformations with sulfasalazine exposure, it is difficult to determine whether the malformations were due to the drug itself or to a combination of factors.[157] Sulfasalazine is a folic acid antagonist and its use should be accompanied by folic acid supplementation.[63]

Antimalarials

Chloroquine exposure in the first trimester at the dosages needed to treat rheumatic diseases has resulted in fetal sensorineural hearing loss.[158] A systematic review in 2009 found no differences in the risk of congenital malformation and spontaneous miscarriage between pregnant women who were treated with hydroxychloroquine for autoimmune disorders and those who were not.[159]

Gold salts

Gold thiomalate and auranofin have proved to be teratogenic in animals,[160] although data from human studies have found them to be safe in pregnancy.[161,162] They can be used if disease control is required, possibly with a reduction in frequency and dose.

Penicillamine salts

Penicillamine salts cross the placenta and there are reports of generalised connective tissue defects such as Ehlers–Danlos syndrome with penicillamine use in pregnancy.[163,164] Another study demonstrated that penicillamine use in pregnancy provides fetal protection against excessive maternal copper levels.[165] The use of penicillamine salts should be limited to conditions where the maternal benefit outweighs the risks.

Corticosteroids

When taken at dosages required for the treatment of rheumatic disorders, no adverse fetal or maternal effects have been reported.[166,167]

Cytotoxic agents

Methotrexate, a folate antagonist, is used frequently for the treatment of rheumatoid arthritis and psoriasis. Methotrexate and alkylating agents such as cyclophosphamide and chlorambucil are considered teratogenic and are likely to cause fetal bone marrow depression, infection and haemorrhage.[168] In addition, there is evidence to suggest an increased risk of miscarriage with methotrexate use in the first trimester.[169] Folic acid supplementation is recommended with methotrexate, and conception should be avoided for 3 months after stopping the treatment.

Cyclophosphamide is given in severe cases of systemic lupus erythematosus nephropathy and immune vasculitis. The risk of congenital malformations with cyclophosphamide use is as high as 16–22%.[170] Again, its use is reserved for cases where the maternal benefit outweighs fetal risk.

Ciclosporin

Ciclosporin is a fungal metabolite and a potent immunosuppressant. Data on the safety of ciclosporin in pregnancy are primarily from renal transplant patients. Case reports on its use in lupus nephritis also confirm its safety in pregnancy.[171]

Treatment of inflammatory bowel disease

In women inflammatory bowel disease is more common during the childbearing years and more women with known disease are presenting to clinics.

5-aminosalicylic acid

5-aminosalicylic acid (5-ASA) has limited systemic absorption and limited transplacental transfer.[172] In a cohort of 146 women exposed to 5-ASA in the first trimester, there was no increase in the rate of major malformations.[173] In a recent meta-analysis of women with inflammatory bowel disease treated with 5-ASA, there was a statistically non-significant increase in the risk of congenital abnormalities (OR 1.16) and spontaneous miscarriage (OR 1.14).[174]

Sulfasalazine

Refer to the section on treatment of rheumatic diseases for information on the use of sulfasalazine in pregnancy (page 107).

Corticosteroids

Corticosteroids can be used both orally and topically (suppositories and enemas) for the treatment of inflammatory bowel disease in pregnancy.

Azathioprine and 6-mercaptopurine

Conflicting reports exist for the use of azathioprine and 6-mercaptopurine in pregnancy. Some studies have shown an increased risk of major congenital defects,[175,176] whereas others have confirmed their safety when used in pregnancy.[177,178] As the benefits of continuing the treatment outweigh the risks, women on azathioprine should not discontinue the drug on becoming pregnant; instead, they should be regularly monitored for signs of myelosuppression.

Infliximab

Data on the use of infliximab in pregnancy are available only from case series and post-marketing surveys.[179,180] There is limited evidence regarding the safety of infliximab in pregnancy and its use should be avoided.

Anti-asthmatics

Asthma is a relatively common condition in pregnant women, with varying severity. Drug treatment is no different from that in non-pregnant women. Few women with asthma require oral corticosteroids: most are on inhaled corticosteroids. Data on oral corticosteroids use in pregnancy confirm its safety (refer to the section on antiemetics for more information on the use of corticosteroids in pregnancy, page 90). Beclomethasone is one of the oldest inhaled corticosteroids and studies have shown no increase in the risk of congenital malformations or adverse fetal effects with its use.[181,182] Other drugs, such as disodium cromoglycate and nedocromil, are also safe for use in early pregnancy.[183] Methylxanthines are used infrequently for the treatment of asthma. Animal studies have shown teratogenic effects, although human data have shown no increase in teratogenicity.[184,185]

Treatment of liver diseases

Hepatitis A and B vaccines can be administered in pregnancy if required. Lamivudine use in hepatitis B is not associated with an increased risk of teratogenicity; only limited data are available for adefovir and entecavir. Interferon and ribavirin are contraindicated for the treatment of active hepatitis C in pregnancy. Ursodeoxycholic acid can be used in pregnant women with primary liver disease if a therapeutic benefit has been confirmed.

Drugs of abuse

Illicit drug use in woman aged 15–35 years is on the rise. Approximately 20% of drug addicts entering treatment are women, and every year as many as 6.5–11% of women who are problem drug users fall pregnant or give birth.[186]

Opioids (heroin)

Opiods are the most commonly misused drugs, and heroin use is the most frequently reported.[187] Heroin is commonly smoked or injected. There is no evidence of teratogenesis with the use of opioids, but they are associated with increased perinatal morbidity and mortality.

Methadone

Methadone is prescribed as a substitute for opioid dependency. Medically, it is preferable to heroin as it is a purer form and can be prescribed as a linctus. Its long half-life and duration of action (greater than 24 hours) make it suitable as substitution therapy.

Buprenorphine

This is a partial opiate agonist with similar effects to heroin use.

Benzodiazepines

Benzodiazepines are often used in association with cocaine to reduce the depressant effects. There are reports of congenital malformations (pyloric stenosis and cardiac and craniofacial defects) with benzodiazepine use in the first trimester of pregnancy.[188,189] In a meta-analysis of cohort studies, no such association was observed (see section on anti-epileptics for more information, page 97).

Amphetamines

Amphetamines are used as stimulants and can be swallowed, smoked or injected. There are no specific effects associated with their use in pregnancy.

Cocaine

Cocaine misuse is harmful in pregnancy. It is injected or snorted/sniffed. Evidence suggests an increased risk of congenital malformations (limb reduction defects and non-duodenal intestinal atresia)[190] and miscarriages[191] with its use in early pregnancy. It is a powerful vasoconstrictor which may cause vascular compromise and adverse effects in the fetus.

Cannabis and d-lysergic acid diethylamide (LSD)

No specific adverse fetal effects have been reported with the use of cannabis and LSD in early pregnancy.

Management of patients with drug exposure

In the emergency gynaecology setting, if a woman has a history of exposure to drugs of misuse in early pregnancy, she should be appropriately counselled in a non-judgemental manner and screened for potential infections. Her antenatal care should be arranged within a multidisciplinary team.

Women with drug exposure in early pregnancy must receive accurate information, as unrealistic perceptions of teratogenic risk may lead to inadequate treatment of maternal disease or termination of an otherwise wanted pregnancy. Management involves providing evidence-based information and counselling.[192]

References

1 Headley J, Northstone K, Simmons H, Golding J. Medication use during pregnancy: data from the Avon Longitudinal Study of Parents and Children. *Eur J Clin Pharmacol* 2004;60:355–61.

2 Macara LM. Identifying fetal abnormalities. In: Rubin P, editor. *Prescribing in Pregnancy*. 3rd ed. London: BMJ Publishing Group; 2000. p. 1–14.

3 Joint Formulary Committee. *British National Formulary*. 57th ed. London: British Medical Association and Royal Pharmaceutical Society of Great Britain; 2009 [www.bnf.org].

4 United States Food and Drug Administration. Labeling and prescription drug advertising. Content and format for labeling for human prescription drugs. *Fed Reg* 1979;44: 434–67.

5 Moore K L. *The Developing Human*. 4th ed. Philadelphia: WB Saunders; 1988.

6 Bentley T G, Willett W C, Weinstein M C, Kuntz K M. Population-level changes in folate intake by age, gender, and race/ethnicity after folic acid fortification. *Am J Public Health* 2006;96:2040–7.

7 Wolff T, Witkop C T, Miller T, Syed S B; U.S. Preventive Services Task Force. Folic acid supplementation for the prevention of neural tube defects: an update of the evidence for the U.S. Preventive Services Task Force. *Ann Intern Med* 2009;150:632–9.

8 Mills J L, Von Kohorn I, Conley M R, Zeller J A, Cox C, Williamson RE, et al. Low vitamin B-12 concentrations in patients without anemia: the effect of folic acid fortification of grain. *Am J Clin Nutr* 2003;77:1474–7.

9 National Collaborating Centre for Women's and Children's Health. *Antenatal care: routine care for the healthy pregnant woman*. London: RCOG Press; 2008. p. 85–6.

10 Gadsby R, Barnie-Adshead A M, Jagger C. A prospective study of nausea and vomiting during pregnancy. *Br J Gen Pract* 1993;43:245–8.

11 Jewell D, Young G. Interventions for nausea and vomiting in early pregnancy. *Cochrane Database Syst Rev* 2003;(4):CD000145.

12 McBride W G. Thalidomide embryopathy. *Teratology* 1977;16:79–82.

13 Seto A, Einarson T, Koren G. Pregnancy outcome following first trimester exposure to antihistamines: meta-analysis. *Am J Perinatol* 1997;14:119–24.

14 Schwarz E B, Moretti M E, Nayak S, Koren G. Risk of hypospadias in offsprig of women using loratadine during pregnancy: a systematic review and meta-analysis. *Drug Saf* 2008;31:775–88.

15 Nelson-Piercy C. Treatment of nausea and vomiting in pregnancy. When should it be treated and what can be safely taken? *Drug Saf* 1998;19:155–64.

16 Gill S K, Einarson A. The safety of drugs for the treatment of nausea and vomiting of pregnancy. *Expert Opin Drug Saf* 2007;6:685–94.

17 Magee L A, Mazzotta P, Koren G. Evidence-based view of safety and effectiveness of pharmacologic therapy for nausea and vomiting of pregnancy (NVP). *Am J Obstet Gynecol* 2002;186 Suppl 5:S256–61.

18 Wilde M I, Markham A. Ondansetron. A review of its pharmacology and preliminary clinical findings in novel applications. *Drugs* 1996;52:773–94.

19 Siu S S, Chan M T, Lau T K. Placental transfer of ondansetron during early human pregnancy. *Clin Pharmacokinet* 2006;45:419–23.

20 Einarson A, Maltepe C, Navioz Y, Kennedy D, Tan M P, Koren G. The safety of ondansetron for nausea and vomiting of pregnancy: a prospective comparative study. *BJOG* 2004;111:940–3.

21 World M J. Ondansetron and hyperemesis gravidarum. *Lancet* 1993;341:185.

22 Siu S S, Yip S K, Cheung C W, Lau T K. Treatment of intractable hyperemesis gravidarum by ondansetron. *Eur J Obstet Gynecol Reprod Biol* 2002;105:73–4.

23 Sullivan C A, Johnson C A, Roach H, Martin R W, Stewart D K, Morrison J C. A pilot study of intravenous ondansetron for hyperemesis gravidarum. *Am J Obstet Gynecol* 1996;174:1565–8.

24 Bracken M Enkin M, Campbell H, Chalmers I. Symptoms in pregnancy: nausea and vomiting, heartburn, constipation, and leg cramps. In: Chalmers I, Enkin M, Keirse M JNC, editors. *Effective Care in Pregnancy and Childbirth*. Oxford: Oxford University Press; 1989. p. 501–11.

25 Mazzotta P, Magee L A. A risk–benefit assessment of pharmacological and nonpharmacological treatments for nausea and vomiting of pregnancy. *Drugs* 2000;59:781–800.

26 Sahakian V, Rouse D, Sipes S, Rose N, Niebyl J. Vitamin B6 is effective therapy for nausea and vomiting of pregnancy: a randomized, double-blind placebo-controlled study. *Obstet Gynecol* 1991;78:33–6.

27 Vutyavanich T, Wongtra-ngan S, Ruangsri R. Pyridoxine for nausea and vomiting of pregnancy: a randomized, double-blind, placebo-controlled trial. *Am J Obstet Gynecol* 1995;173:881–4.

28 Brent R L. Bendectin: review of the medical literature of a comprehensively studied human nonteratogen and the most prevalent tortogen-litigen. *Reprod Toxicol* 1995;9:337–49.

29 Ziaei S, Hosseiney FS, Faghihzadeh S. The efficacy low dose of prednisolone in the treatment of hyperemesis gravidarum. *Acta Obstet Gynecol Scand* 2004;83:272–5.

30 Nelson-Piercy C, Fayers P, de Swiet M. Randomised, double-blind, placebo-controlled trial of corticosteroids for the treatment of hyperemesis gravidarum. *BJOG* 2001;108:9–15.

31 Bondok R S, El Sharnouby N M, Eid H E, Abd Elmaksoud A M. Pulsed steroid therapy is an effective treatment for intractable hyperemesis gravidarum. *Crit Care Med* 2006;34:2781–3.

32 Marrero J M, Goggin P M, de Caestecker J S, Pearce J M, Maxwell J D. Determinants of pregnancy heartburn. *Br J Obstet Gynaecol* 1992;99:731–4.

33 Association of the British Pharmaceutical Industry. *ABPI Compendium of Data Sheets and Summaries of Product Characteristics*. London: Datapharm Communications; 2001.

34 Rayburn W, Liles E, Christensen H, Robinson M. Antacids vs. antacids plus non-prescription ranitidine for heartburn during pregnancy. *Int J Gynaecol Obstet* 1999;66:35–7.

35 Magee L A, Inocencion G, Kamboj L, Rosetti F, Koren G. Safety of first trimester exposure to histamine H2 blockers. A prospective cohort study. *Dig Dis Sci* 1996;41:1145–9.

36 Parker S, Schade R R, Pohl C R, Gavaler J S, Van Thiel D H. Prenatal and neonatal exposure of male rat pups to cimetidine but not ranitidine adversely affects subsequent adult sexual functioning. *Gastroenterology* 1984;86:675–80.

37 Lalkin A, Loebstein R, Addis A, Ramezani-Namin F, Mastroiacovo P, Mazzone T, et al. The safety of omeprazole during pregnancy: a multicenter prospective controlled study. *Am J Obstet Gynecol* 1998;179:727–30.

38 Nikfar S, Abdollahi M, Moretti M E, Magee L A, Koren G. Use of proton pump inhibitors during pregnancy and rates of major malformations: a meta-analysis. *Dig Dis Sci* 2002; 47:1526–9.

39 National Collaborating Centre for Women's and Children's Health. *Antenatal care: routine care for the healthy pregnant woman*. London: RCOG Press; 2008. p. 109.

40 Streissguth A P, Treder R P, Barr H M, Shepard T H, Bleyer W A, Sampson PD, et al. Aspirin and acetaminophen use by pregnant women and subsequent child IQ and attention decrements. *Teratology* 1987;35:211–19.

41 CLASP: a randomised trial of low-dose aspirin for the prevention and treatment of pre-eclampsia among 9364 pregnant women. CLASP (Collaborative Low-dose Aspirin Study in Pregnancy) Collaborative Group. *Lancet* 1994;343:619–29.

42 Buckfield P. Major congenital faults in newborn infants: a pilot study in New Zealand. *N Z Med J* 1973;78:195–204.

43 Turner G, Collins E. Fetal effects of regular salicylate ingestion in pregnancy. *Lancet* 1975;2:338–9.

44 Slone D, Siskind V, Heinonen OP, Monson RR, Kaufman DW, Shapiro S. Aspirin and congenital malformations. *Lancet* 1976;1:1373–5.

45 Byron MA. Treatment of rheumatic diseases. *Br Med J (Clin Res Ed)* 1987;294:236–8.

46 Briggs G G, Freeman R K, Yaffe S J. *Drugs in pregnancy and lactation: a reference guide to fetal and neonatal risk.* 5th ed. Baltimore/London: Williams & Wilkins; 1998.

47 Marcus D A, Scharff L, Turk D. Longitudinal prospective study of headache during pregnancy and postpartum. *Headache* 1999;39:625–32.

48 Sances G, Granella F, Nappi R E, Fignon A, Ghiotto N, Polatti F, et al. Course of migraine during pregnancy and postpartum: a prospective study. *Cephalalgia* 2003;23: 197–205.

49 Graham JM Jr, Marin-Padilla M, Hoefnagel D. Jejunal atresia associated with Cafergot ingestion during pregnancy. *Clin Pediatr (Phila)* 1983;22:226–8.

50 Hughes H E, Goldstein D A. Birth defects following maternal exposure to ergotamine, beta blockers, and caffeine. *J Med Genet* 1988;25:396–9.

51 Graf W D, Shepard T H. Uterine contraction in the development of Möbius syndrome. *J Child Neurol* 1997; 12:225–7.

52 Fenster L, Hubbard A E, Swan S H, Windham G C, Waller K, Hiatt RA, et al. Caffeinated beverages, decaffeinated coffee, and spontaneous abortion. *Epidemiology* 1997;8:515–23.

53 Cnattingius S, Signorello LB, Annerén G, Clausson B, Ekbom A, Ljunger E, et al. Caffeine intake and the risk of first-trimester spontaneous abortion. *N Engl J Med* 2000;343:1839–45.

54 Hardebo J E, Edvinsson L. Reduced sensitivity to alpha- and beta-adrenergic receptor agonists of intra- and extracranial vessels during pregnancy. Relevance to migraine. *Acta Neurol Scand Suppl* 1977;64:204–5.

55 Schenker S, Yang Y, Perez A, Henderson GI, Lee M P. Sumatriptan (Imitrex) transport by the human placenta. *Proc Soc Exp Biol Med* 1995;210:213–20.

56 Fox A W, Chambers C D, Anderson P O, Diamond M L, Spierings E L. Evidence-based assessment of pregnancy outcome after sumatriptan exposure. *Headache* 2002;42: 8–15.

57 Dalton I. A (H1N1) swine influenza: phase two of the vaccination programme. Department of Health. London: Richmond House; 2009 [www.dh.gov.uk/en/Publicationsandstatistics/Lettersandcirculars/Dearcolleagueletters/DH_108844].

58 Mastroiacovo P, Mazzone T, Botto L D, Serafini M A, Finardi A, Caramelli L, et al. Prospective assessment of pregnancy outcomes after first-trimester exposure to fluconazole. *Am J Obstet Gynecol* 1996;175:1645–50.

59 Pursley T J, Blomquist I K, Abraham J, Andersen H F, Bartley J A. Fluconazole-induced congenital anomalies in three infants. *Clin Infect Dis* 1996;22:336–40.

60 Brocklehurst P, Rooney G. Interventions for treating genital chlamydia trachomatis infection in pregnancy. *Cochrane Database Syst Rev* 2000;(4):CD 000054.

61 Peterson H B, Walker C K, Kahn J G, Washington A E, Eschenbach D A, Faro S. Pelvic inflammatory disease. Key treatment issues and options. *JAMA* 1991;266:2605–11.

62 Bar-Oz B, Moretti M E, Boskovic R, O'Brien L, Koren G. The safety of quinolones—a meta-analysis of pregnancy outcomes. *Eur J Obstet Gynecol Reprod Biol* 2009;143:75–8.

63 Hernández-Díaz S, Werler M M, Walker A M, Mitchell A A. Neural tube defects in relation to use of folic acid antagonists during pregnancy. *Am J Epidemiol* 2001;153:961–8.

64 Sivojelezova A, Einarson A, Shuhaiber S, Koren G; Motherisk Team. Trimethoprim-sulfonamide combination therapy in early pregnancy. *Can Fam Physician* 2003;49: 1085–6.

65 Einarson A, Shuhaiber S, Koren G. Effects of antibacterials on the unborn child: what is known and how should this influence prescribing. *Paediatr Drugs* 2001;3:803–16.

66 Ormerod L P. Tuberculosis screening and prevention in new immigrants 1983–88. *Respir Med* 1990;84:269–71.

67 Assael B M, Parini R, Rusconi F. Ototoxicity of aminoglycoside antibiotics in infants and children. *Pediatr Infect Dis* 1982;1:357–65.

68 Ullberg S, Lindquist N G, Sjöstrand S E. Accumulation of chorio-retinotoxic drugs in the foetal eye. *Nature* 1970;227:1257–8.

69 Lewis R, Lauersen N H, Birnbaum S. Malaria associated with pregnancy. *Obstet Gynecol* 1973;42:696–700.

70 Bradley D J, Warhurst D C. Guidelines for the prevention of malaria in travellers from the United Kingdom. PHLS Malaria Reference Laboratory, London School of Hygiene and Tropical Medicine. *Commun Dis Rep CDR Rev* 1997;7:R137–52.

71 de Ruiter A, Mercey D, Anderson J, Chakraborty R, Clayden P, Foster G, et al. British HIV Association and Children's HIV Association guidelines for the management of HIV infection in pregnant women 2008. *HIV Med* 2008;9:452–502.

72 Shaffer N, Chuachoowong R, Mock P A, Bhadrakom C, Siriwasin W, Young N L, et al. Short-course zidovudine for perinatal HIV-1 transmission in Bangkok, Thailand: a randomised controlled trial. Bangkok Collaborative Perinatal HIV Transmission Study Group. *Lancet* 1999;353:773–80.

73 Connor E M, Sperling R S, Gelber R, Kiselev P, Scott G, O'Sullivan M J, et al. Reduction of maternal–infant transmission of human immunodeficiency virus type 1 with zidovudine treatment. Pediatric AIDS Clinical Trials Group Protocol 076 Study Group. *N Engl J Med* 1994;331:1173–80.

74 Lallemant M, Jourdain G, Le Coeur S, Kim S, Koetsawang S, Comeau A M, et al. A trial of shortened zidovudine regimens to prevent mother-to-child transmission of human immunodeficiency virus type 1. Perinatal HIV Prevention Trial (Thailand) Investigators. *N Engl J Med* 2000;343:982–91.

75 Mayaux M J, Teglas J P, Mandelbrot L, Berrebi A, Gallais H, Matheron S, et al. Acceptability and impact of zidovudine for prevention of mother-to-child human immunodeficiency virus-1 transmission in France. *J Pediatr* 1997;131:857–62.

76 Wade N A, Birkhead G S, Warren B L, Charbonneau T T, French P T, Wang L, et al. Abbreviated regimens of zidovudine prophylaxis and perinatal transmission of the human immunodeficiency virus. *N Engl J Med* 1998;339:1409–14.

77 Pennell P B. Pregnancy in women who have epilepsy. *Neurol Clin* 2004;22:799–820.

78 Motamedi G K, Meador K J. Antiepileptic drugs and neurodevelopment. *Curr Neurol Neurosci Rep* 2006;6:341–6.

79 Pennell P B. The importance of monotherapy in pregnancy. *Neurology* 2003;60 Suppl 4:S31–8.

80 Meador K J, Baker G A, Finnell R H, Kalayjian L A, Liporace J D, Loring D W, et al. In utero antiepileptic drug exposure: fetal death and malformations. *Neurology* 2006;67:407–12.

81 Holmes L B, Wyszynski D F, Lieberman E. The AED (antiepileptic drug) pregnancy registry: a 6-year experience. *Arch Neurol* 2004;61:673–8.

82 Finnell R H, Nau H, Yerby M S. General principles: teratogenicity of antiepileptic drugs. In: Levy R H, Matson B S, editors. *Antiepileptic drugs*. New York: Raven Press; 1995. p. 209–30.

83 Hanson J W, Smith D W. The fetal hydantoin syndrome. *J Pediatr* 1975;87:285–90.

84 Jones K L, Lacro R V, Johnson K A, Adams J. Pattern of malformations in the children of women treated with carbamazepine during pregnancy. *N Engl J Med* 1989;320:1661–6.

85 Jones K L, Johnson K A, Chambers C C. Pregnancy outcome in women treated with phenobarbital monotherapy. *Teratology* 1992;45:453–54.

86 Wilkie A O, Morriss-Kay G M. Genetics of craniofacial development and malformation. *Nat Rev Genet* 2001;2: 458–68.

87 Bjerkedal T, Czeizel A, Goujard J, Kallen B, Mastroiacova P, Nevin N, et al. Valproic acid and spina bifida. *Lancet* 1982; 2:1096.

88 Wide K, Winbladh B, Källén B. Major malformations in infants exposed to antiepileptic drugs in utero, with emphasis on carbamazepine and valproic acid: a nation-wide, population-based register study. *Acta Paediatr* 2004;93:174–6.

89 Artama M, Auvinen A, Raudaskoski T, Isojarvi I, Isojärvi J. Antiepileptic drug use of women with epilepsy and congenital malformations in offspring. *Neurology* 2005;64:1874–8.

90 Fedrick J. Epilepsy and pregnancy: a report from the Oxford Record Linkage Study. *Br Med J* 1973;2:442–8.

91 Lindhout D, Omtzigt J G. Teratogenic effects of antiepileptic drugs: implications for the management of epilepsy in women of childbearing age. *Epilepsia* 1994;35 Suppl 4:S19–28.

92 Montouris G. Safety of the newer antiepileptic drug oxocarbazepine during pregnancy. *Curr Med Res Opin* 2005;21:693–701.

93 Dolovich L R, Addis A, Vaillancourt J M, Power J D, Koren G, Einarson T R. Benzodiazepine use in pregnancy and major malformations or oral cleft: meta-analysis of cohort and case–control studies. *BMJ* 1998;317:839–43.

94 Cunnington M, Ferber S, Quartey G; International Lamotrigine Pregnancy Registry Scientific Advisory Committee. Effect of dose on the frequency of major birth defects following fetal exposure to lamotrigine monotherapy in an international observational study. *Epilepsia* 2007;48:1207–10.

95 Yerby M S. Management issues for women with epilepsy: neural tube defects and folic acid supplementation. *Neurology* 2003;61 Suppl 2:S23–6.

96 Saftlas A F, Olson D R, Franks A L, Atrash H K, Pokras R. Epidemiology of preeclampsia and eclampsia in the United States, 1979–1986. *Am J Obstet Gynecol* 1990;163:460–5.

97 Hytten F, Chamberlain G. *Clinical Physiology in Obstetrics.* Boston: Blackwell Scientific Publications; 1980.

98 Redman C W, Beilin L J, Bonnar J. Treatment of hypertension in pregnancy with methyldopa: blood pressure control and side effects. *Br J Obstet Gynaecol* 1977;84: 419–26.

99 Jones H M, Cummings A J, Setchell K D, Lawson A M. A study of the disposition of alpha-methyldopa in newborn infants following its administration to the mother for the treatment of hypertension during pregnancy. *Br J Clin Pharmacol* 1979;8:433–40.

100 Ounsted M, Cockburn J, Moar V A, Redman C W. Maternal hypertension with superimposed pre-eclampsia: effects on child development at 7½ years. *Br J Obstet Gynaecol* 1983;90:644–9.

101 Isaac L. Clonidine in the central nervous system: site and mechanism of hypotensive action. *J Cardiovasc Pharmacol* 1980;2 Suppl 1:S5–19.

102 Butters L, Kennedy S, Rubin P C. Atenolol in essential hypertension during pregnancy. *BMJ* 1990;301:587–9.

103 Lip G Y, Beevers M, Churchill D, Shaffer L M, Beevers D G. Effect of atenolol on birth weight. *Am J Cardiol* 1997;79:1436–8.

104 Dubois D, Petitcolas J, Temperville B, Klepper A, Catherine P. Treatment of hypertension in pregnancy with beta-adrenoceptor antagonists. *Br J Clin Pharmacol* 1982;13 Suppl 2:375S–8.

105 Fidler J, Smith V, Fayers P, de Swiet M. Randomised controlled comparative study of methyldopa and oxprenolol in treatment of hypertension in pregnancy. *Br Med J (Clin Res Ed)* 1983;286:1927–30.

106 Plouin P F, Breart G, Maillard F, Papiernik E, Relier J P. Comparison of antihypertensive efficacy and perinatal safety of labetalol and methyldopa in the treatment of hypertension in pregnancy: a randomized controlled trial. *Br J Obstet Gynaecol* 1988;95:868–76.

107 Pickles C J, Symonds E M, Broughton Pipkin F. The fetal outcome in a randomized double-blind controlled trial of labetalol versus placebo in pregnancy-induced hypertension. *Br J Obstet Gynaecol* 1989;96:38–43.

108 Kanto J H. Current status of labetalol, the first alpha- and beta-blocking agent. *Int J Clin Pharmacol Ther Toxicol* 1985;23:617–28.

109 Magee L A, Schick B, Donnenfeld A E, Sage S R, Conover B, Cook L, et al. The safety of calcium channel blockers in human pregnancy: a prospective, multicenter cohort study. *Am J Obstet Gynecol* 1996;174:823–8.

110 Knott P D, Thorpe S S, Lamont C A. Congenital renal dysgenesis possibly due to captopril. *Lancet* 1989;1:451.

111 Kreft-Jais C, Plouin P F, Tchobroutsky C, Boutroy M J. Angiotensin-converting enzyme inhibitors during pregnancy: a survey of 22 patients given captopril and nine given enalapril. *Br J Obstet Gynaecol* 1988;95:420–2.

112 Martin R A, Jones K L, Mendoza A, Barr M Jr, Benirschke K. Effect of ACE inhibition on the fetal kidney: decreased renal blood flow. *Teratology* 1992;46:317–21.

113 Lip G Y, Churchill D, Beevers M, Auckett A, Beevers D G. Angiotensin-converting-enzyme inhibitors in early pregnancy. *Lancet* 1997;350:1446–7.

114 Centers for Disease Control and Prevention. Postmarketing surveillance for angiotensin-converting enzyme inhibitor use during the first trimester of pregnancy—United States, Canada, and Israel, 1987–1995. *JAMA* 1997;277:1193–4.

115 Steffensen F H, Nielsen G L, Sørensen H T, Olesen C, Olsen J. Pregnancy outcome with ACE-inhibitor use in early pregnancy. *Lancet* 1998;351:596.

116 Sibai B M, Anderson G D, Spinnato J A, Shaver D C. Plasma volume findings in patients with mild pregnancy-induced hypertension. *Am J Obstet Gynecol* 1983;147:16–19.

117 Collins R, Yusuf S, Peto R. Overview of randomised trials of diuretics in pregnancy. *Br Med J (Clin Res Ed)* 1985;290: 17–23.

118 Report of the Canadian Hypertension Society Consensus Conference: 3. Pharmacologic treatment of hypertensive disorders in pregnancy. *CMAJ* 1997;157:1245–54.

119 Viguera A C, Whitfield T, Baldessarini R J, Newport D J, Stowe Z, Reminick A, et al. Risk of recurrence in women with bipolar disorder during pregnancy: prospective study of mood stabilizer discontinuation. *Am J Psychiatry* 2007;164:1817–24.

120 Webb R T, Howard L, Abel K M. Antipsychotic drugs for non-affective psychosis during pregnancy and postpartum. *Cochrane Database Syst Rev* 2004;(2):CD004411.

121 Cohen L S, Rosenbaum J F. Psychotropic drug use during pregnancy: weighing the risks. *J Clin Psychiatry* 1998;59 Suppl 2:18–28.

122 Baum A L, Misri S. Selective serotonin-reuptake inhibitors in pregnancy and lactation. *Harv Rev Psychiatry* 1996;4:117–25.

123 Mourilhe P, Stokes P E. Risks and benefits of selective serotonin reuptake inhibitors in the treatment of depression. *Drug Saf* 1998;18:57–82.

124 Bar-Oz B, Einarson T, Einarson A, Boskovic R, O'Brien L, Malm H, et al. Paroxetine and congenital malformations: meta-analysis and consideration of potential confounding factors. *Clin Ther* 2007;29:918–26.

125 Davis R L, Rubanowice D, McPhillips H, Raebel M A, Andrade S E, Smith D, et al. Risks of congenital malformations and perinatal events among infants exposed to antidepressant medications during pregnancy. *Pharmacoepidemiol Drug Saf* 2007;16:1086–94.

126 O'Brien L, Einarson T R, Sarkar M, Einarson A, Koren G. Does paroxetine cause cardiac malformations? *J Obstet Gynaecol Can* 2008;30:696–701.

127 Cohen L S, Friedman J M, Jefferson J W, Johnson E M, Weiner M L. A reevaluation of risk of in utero exposure to lithium. *JAMA* 1994;271:146–50.

128 Mander A J, Loudon J B. Rapid recurrence of mania following abrupt discontinuation of lithium. *Lancet* 1988;2:15–17.

129 Pinkofsky H B. Psychosis during pregnancy: treatment considerations. *Ann Clin Psychiatry* 1997;9:175–9.

130 Altshuler L L, Cohen L, Szuba M P, Burt V K, Gitlin M, Mintz J. Pharmacologic management of psychiatric illness during pregnancy: dilemmas and guidelines. *Am J Psychiatry* 1996;153:592–606.

131 Inoue M, Arata N, Koren G, Ito S. Hyperthyroidism during pregnancy. *Can Fam Physician* 2009;55:701–3.

132 Girling J C, de Swiet M. Thyroxine dosage during pregnancy in women with primary hypothyroidism. *Br J Obstet Gynaecol* 1992;99:368–70.

133 Neale D, Burrow G. Thyroid disease in pregnancy. *Obstet Gynecol Clin North Am* 2004;31:893–905, xi.

134 Clementi M, Di Gianantonio E, Pelo E, Mammi I, Basile RT, Tenconi R. Methimazole embryopathy: delineation of the phenotype. *Am J Med Genet* 1999;83:43–6.

135 Barbero P, Ricagni C, Mercado G, Bronberg R, Torrado M. Choanal atresia associated with prenatal methimazole exposure: three new patients. *Am J Med Genet A* 2004;129A:83–6.

136 Martínez-Frías M L, Cereijo A, Rodríguez-Pinilla E, Urioste M. Methimazole in animal feed and congenital aplasia cutis. *Lancet* 1992;339:742–3.

137 Di Gianantonio E, Schaefer C, Mastroiacovo PP, Cournot MP, Benedicenti F, Reuvers M, et al. Adverse effects of prenatal methimazole exposure. *Teratology* 2001;64:262–6.

138 Wing D A, Millar L K, Koonings P P, Montoro M N, Mestman J H. A comparison of propylthiouracil versus methimazole in the treatment of hyperthyroidism in pregnancy. *Am J Obstet Gynecol* 1994;170:90–5.

139 Confidential Enquiry into Maternal and Child Health. *Pregnancy in women with type 1 and type 2 diabetes in 2002–2003, England, Wales and Northern Ireland.* London: CEMACH; 2005.

140 Gutzin S J, Kozer E, Magee L A, Feig D S, Koren G. The safety of oral hypoglycemic agents in the first trimester of pregnancy: a meta-analysis. *Can J Clin Pharmacol* 2003;10:179–83.

141 Koren G, Gilbert C, Valois M. Metformin use during the first trimester of pregnancy. Is it safe? *Can Fam Physician* 2006;52:171–2.

142 Ekpebegh C O, Coetzee E J, van der Merwe L, Levitt N S. A 10-year retrospective analysis of pregnancy outcome in pregestational type 2 diabetes: comparison of insulin and oral glucose-lowering agents. *Diabet Med* 2007;24:253–8.

143 P Krupp, Turkalj I. Surveillance of Parlodel (bromocriptine) in pregnancy and offspring. In: Jacobs H, editor. *Prolactinomas and Pregnancy.* Lancaster: MTP Press; 1984: p. 45–50.

144 Bigazzi M, Ronga R, Lancranjan I, Ferraro S, Branconi F, Buzzoni P, et al. A pregnancy in an acromegalic woman during bromocriptine treatment: effects on growth hormone and prolactin in the maternal, fetal, and amniotic compartments. *J Clin Endocrinol Metab* 1979;48:9–12.

145 Gormley M J, Hadden D R, Kennedy T L, Montgomery D A, Murnaghan G A, Sheridan B. Cushing's syndrome in pregnancy—treatment with metyrapone. *Clin Endocrinol (Oxf)* 1982;16:283–93.

146 Aron D C, Schnall A M, Sheeler L R. Cushing's syndrome and pregnancy. *Am J Obstet Gynecol* 1990;162:244–52.

147 Melissari E, Parker C J, Wilson N V, Monte G, Kanthou C, Pemberton K D, et al. Use of low molecular weight heparin in pregnancy. *Thromb Haemost* 1992;68:652–6.

148 Abbott A, Sibert J R, Weaver J B. Chondrodysplasia punctata and maternal warfarin treatment. *Br Med J* 1977;1:1639–40.

149 Shaul W L, Hall J G. Multiple congenital anomalies associated with oral anticoagulants. *Am J Obstet Gynecol* 1977;127:191–8.

150 Chen W W, Chan C S, Lee P K, Wang R Y, Wong V C. Pregnancy in patients with prosthetic heart valves: an experience with 45 pregnancies. *Q J Med* 1982;51:358–65.

151 Iturbe-Alessio I, Fonseca M C, Mutchinik O, Santos M A, Zajarias A, Salazar E. Risks of anticoagulant therapy in pregnant women with artificial heart valves. *N Engl J Med* 1986;315:1390–3.

152 Saour J N, Sieck J O, Mamo L A, Gallus A S. Trial of different intensities of anticoagulation in patients with prosthetic heart valves. *N Engl J Med* 1990;322:428–32.

153 de Swiet M. Anticoagulants. In: Rubin P, editor. *Prescribing in Pregnancy*. 3rd ed. London: BMJ Publishing Group; 2000. p. 47–64.

154 Khan A K, Truelove S C. Placental and mammary transfer of sulphasalazine. *Br Med J* 1979;2:1553.

155 Mogadam M, Dobbins W O 3rd, Korelitz B I, Ahmed S W. Pregnancy in inflammatory bowel disease: effect of sulfasalazine and corticosteroids on fetal outcome. *Gastroenterology* 1981;80:72–6.

156 Nørgård B, Czeizel A E, Rockenbauer M, Olsen J, Sørensen H T. Population-based case control study of the safety of sulfasalazine use during pregnancy. *Aliment Pharmacol Ther* 2001;15:483–6.

157 Craxi A, Pagliarello F. Possible embryotoxicity of sulfasalazine. *Arch Intern Med* 1980;140:1674.

158 Hart C W, Naunton R F. The ototoxicity of chloroquine phosphate. *Arch Otolaryngol* 1964;80:407–12.

159 Sperber K, Hom C, Chao C P, Shapiro D, Ash J. Systematic review of hydroxychloroquine use in pregnant patients with autoimmune diseases. *Pediatr Rheumatol Online J* 2009;7:9.

160 Brooks P M, Needs C J. Antirheumatic drugs in pregnancy and lactation. *Baillieres Clin Rheumatol* 1990;4:157–71.

161 Cohen D L, Orzel J, Taylor A. Infants of mothers receiving gold therapy. *Arthritis Rheum* 1981;24:104–5.

162 Ostensen M, Husby G. Antirheumatic drug treatment during pregnancy and lactation. *Scand J Rheumatol* 1985;14:1–7.

163 Mjolnerod O K, Dommerud S A, Rasmussen K, Gjeruldsen S T. Congenital connective-tissue defect probably due to D-penicillamine treatment in pregnancy. *Lancet* 1971;1:673–5.

164 Solomon L, Abrams G, Dinner M, Berman L. Neonatal abnormalities associated with D-penicillamine treatment during pregnancy. *N Engl J Med* 1977;296:54–5.

165 Scheinberg I H, Sternlieb I. Pregnancy in penicillamine-treated patients with Wilson's disease. *N Engl J Med* 1975;293:1300–2.

166 Popert A J. Pregnancy and adrenocortical hormones. Some aspects of their interaction in rheumatic diseases. *Br Med J* 1962;1:967–72.

167 Grigor R R, Shervington P C, Hughes G R, Hawkins D F. Outcome of pregnancy in systemic lupus erythematosus. *Proc R Soc Med* 1977;70:99–100.

168 Barber H R. Fetal and neonatal effects of cytotoxic agents. *Obstet Gynecol* 1981;58:41S–7S.

169 Kozlowski R D, Steinbrunner J V, MacKenzie A H, Clough J D, Wilke W S, Segal A M. Outcome of first-trimester exposure to low-dose methotrexate in eight patients with rheumatic disease. *Am J Med* 1990;88:589–92.

170 Roubenoff R, Hoyt J, Petri M, Hochberg M C, Hellmann D B. Effects of antiinflammatory and immunosuppressive drugs on pregnancy and fertility. *Semin Arthritis Rheum* 1988;18:88–110.

171 Hussein M M, Mooij J M, Roujouleh H. Cyclosporine in the treatment of lupus nephritis including two patients treated during pregnancy. *Clin Nephrol* 1993;40:160–3.

172 Tett S E. Clinical pharmacokinetics of slow-acting antirheumatic drugs. *Clin Pharmacokinet* 1993;25:392–407.

173 Diav-Citrin O, Park Y H, Veerasuntharam G, Polachek H, Bologa M, Pastuszak A, et al. The safety of mesalamine in human pregnancy: a prospective controlled cohort study. *Gastroenterology* 1998;114:23–8.

174 Rahimi R, Nikfar S, Rezaie A, Abdollahi M. Pregnancy outcome in women with inflammatory bowel disease following exposure to 5-aminosalicylic acid drugs: a meta-analysis. *Reprod Toxicol* 2008;25:271–5.

175 Cornish J, Tan E, Teare J, Teoh T G, Rai R, Clark S K, et al. A meta-analysis on the influence of inflammatory bowel disease on pregnancy. *Gut* 2007;56:830–7.

176 Norgard B, Pedersen L, Christensen L A, Sorensen H T. Therapeutic drug use in women with Crohn's disease and birth outcomes: a Danish nationwide cohort study. *Am J Gastroenterol* 2007;102:1406–13.

177 Ramsey-Goldman R, Mientus J M, Kutzer J E, Mulvihill J J, Medsger T A Jr. Pregnancy outcome in women with systemic lupus erythematosus treated with immunosuppressive drugs. *J Rheumatol* 1993;20:1152–7.

178 Francella A, Dyan A, Bodian C, Rubin P, Chapman M, Present D H. The safety of 6-mercaptopurine for childbearing patients with inflammatory bowel disease: a retrospective cohort study. *Gastroenterology* 2003;124:9–17.

179 Katz J A, Antoni C, Keenan G F, Smith D E, Jacobs S J, Lichtenstein G R. Outcome of pregnancy in women receiving infliximab for the treatment of Crohn's disease and rheumatoid arthritis. *Am J Gastroenterol* 2004;99:2385–92.

180 Mahadevan U, Kane S, Sandborn W J, Cohen R D, Hanson K, Terdiman J P, et al. Intentional infliximab use during pregnancy for induction or maintenance of remission in Crohn's disease. *Aliment Pharmacol Ther* 2005;21:733–8.

181 Brown H M, Storey G, Jackson F A. Beclomethasone dipropionate aerosol in long-term treatment of perennial and seasonal asthma in children and adults: a report of five-and-half years' experience in 600 asthmatic patients. *Br J Clin Pharmacol* 1977;4:259S–267S.

182 Greenberger P A, Patterson R. Beclomethasone diproprionate for severe asthma during pregnancy. *Ann Intern Med* 1983;98:478–80.

183 Schatz M. Asthma treatment during pregnancy. What can be safely taken? *Drug Saf* 1997;16:342–50.

184 Gyarmathy V A, Giraudon I, Hedrich D, Montanari L, Guarita B, Wiessing L. Drug use and pregnancy – challenges for public health. *Euro Surveill* 2009;14:336.

185 Hepburn M. Drugs of Abuse. In: Rubin P, editor. *Prescribing in Pregnancy*. 3rd ed. London: BMJ Publishing Group; 2000. p. 156–69.

186 Bracken M B, Holford T R. Exposure to prescribed drugs in pregnancy and association with congenital malformations. *Obstet Gynecol* 1981;58:336–44.

187 Laegreid L, Olegård R, Walström J, Conradi N. Teratogenic effects of benzodiazepine use during pregnancy. *J Pediatr* 1989;114:126–31.

188 Bingol N, Fuchs M, Diaz V, Stone R K, Gromisch D S. Teratogenicity of cocaine in humans. *J Pediatr* 1987;110:93–6.

189 Chasnoff I J, Burns W J, Schnoll S H, Burns K A. Cocaine use in pregnancy. *N Engl J Med* 1985;313:666–9.

190 Goodwin J, Rieder S, Rieder M J, Matsui D. Counseling regarding pregnancy-related drug exposures by family physicians in Ontario. *Can J Clin Pharmacol* 2007;14:e58–69.

191 Lammer E J, Chen D T, Hoar R M, Agnish N D, Benke P J, Braun J T, et al. Retinoic acid embryopathy. *N Engl J Med* 1985;313:837–41.

192 Strauss J S, Cunningham W J, Leyden J J, Pochi PE, Shalita A R. Isotretinoin and teratogenicity. *J Am Acad Dermatol* 1988;19:353–4.

193 Warkany J. Aminopterin and methotrexate: folic acid deficiency. *Teratology* 1978;17:353–7.

194 Hall J G, Pauli R M, Wilson K M. Maternal and fetal sequelae of anticoagulation during pregnancy. *Am J Med* 1980;68:122–40.

195 Stevenson R E, Burton O M, Ferlauto G J, Taylor H A. Hazards of oral anticoagulants during pregnancy. *JAMA* 1980;243:1549–51.

196 Herbst A L, Scully R E, Robboy S J. Vaginal adenosis and other diethylstilbestrol-related abnormalities. *Clin Obstet Gynecol* 1975;18:185–94.

197 Sandberg E C, Riffle N L, Higdon J V, Getman C E. Pregnancy outcome in women exposed to diethylstilbestrol in utero. *Am J Obstet Gynecol* 1981;140:194–205.

198 Martin J L, Brown C E, Matthews-Davis N, Reardon J E. Effects of antiviral nucleoside analogs on human DNA polymerases and mitochondrial DNA synthesis. *Antimicrob Agents Chemother* 1994;38:2743–9.

199 Baylor M S, Johann-Liang R. Hepatotoxicity associated with nevirapine use. *J Acquir Immune Defic Syndr* 2004;35:538–9.

200 Eastone J A, Decker C F. New-onset diabetes mellitus associated with use of protease inhibitor. *Ann Intern Med* 1997;127:948.

201 Visnegarwala F, Krause K L, Musher D M. Severe diabetes associated with protease inhibitor therapy. *Ann Intern Med* 1997;127:947.

202 Augenbraun M, Minkoff H L. Antiretroviral therapy in the pregnant woman. *Obstet Gynecol Clin North Am* 1997;24:833–54.

203 National Collaborating Centre for Women's and Children's Health. *Diabetes in pregnancy: management of diabetes and its complications from preconception to the postnatal period.* London: RCOG Press; 2008 [guidance.nice.org.uk/CG63].

9 Diagnosis of tubal ectopic pregnancy

Emma Kirk

Introduction

More than 10,000 ectopic pregnancies are diagnosed annually in the UK.[1] Table 9.1 shows the prevalence and mortality rate for ectopic pregnancies in the UK since 1991. The majority of these ectopic pregnancies (around 95%) occur in the fallopian tube, with the ampullary region of the tube being the most common site for ectopic implantation. According to published data, between 2.3% and 3.9% of women attending early pregnancy units in the UK will be diagnosed with an ectopic pregnancy.[2,3]

Presentation

Women with ectopic pregnancies have been described as presenting with a classic triad of symptoms: pain, vaginal bleeding and a history of amenor-rhoea.[4] These symptoms may be accompanied by shoulder tip pain (a reflec-

TABLE 9.1 **Incidence and mortality rate for ectopic pregnancies in the UK, 1991–2005**

Years	Estimated pregnancies (*n*)	Estimated ectopic pregnancies (*n*)	Rate/1000 pregnancies (95% CI)	Mortality rate/1000 pregnancies (95% CI)
1991–93	3 141 667	30 160	9.6 (9.5–9.7)	0.29 (0.15–0.55)
1994–96	2 917 391	33 550	11.5 (11.4–11.6)	0.41 (0.24–0.72)
1997–99	2 878 012	31 946	11.1 (11.0–11.2)	0.45 (0.26–0.77)
2000–02	2 736 364	30 100	11.0 (10.9–11.1)	0.40 (0.22–0.72)
2003–05	2 891 892	32 100	11.1 (10.9–11.1)	0.35 (0.19–0.64)

tion of significant haemoperitoneum with blood irritating the diaphragm), syncope and shock. Fortunately, in the UK, presentation with these accompanying symptoms is relatively unusual as the majority of ectopic pregnancies are diagnosed earlier in the course of the condition. Home urinary pregnancy tests now enable a pregnancy to be diagnosed even before a menstrual period is missed, so women often present at very early gestations before any symptoms have developed. Women in the UK may also present early because of the existence of early pregnancy units, which often have open access and thus encourage women to attend.

It has been reported that 9% of women with an ectopic pregnancy have no history of pelvic pain[5] and 36% lack adnexal tenderness on pelvic examination.[6] However, atypical presentations are not uncommon. Ectopic pregnancy can mimic other gynaecological disorders and gastrointestinal or urinary tract diseases, such as acute salpingitis, ruptured corpus luteum cyst, ovarian torsion, miscarriage, appendicitis and urinary tract infections. In the 1997–99 Report of the Confidential Enquiries into Maternal Deaths in the United Kingdom it was stated that most of the women who died from ectopic pregnancy were misdiagnosed in the primary care or accident and emergency department setting.[7] The report therefore recommended that all clinicians should be aware of atypical clinical presentations of ectopic pregnancy. A key recommendation of the 2003–05 report was that practitioners should consider ectopic pregnancy in women presenting with diarrhoea and vomiting, after four of the ten women who died from ectopic pregnancy during that triennium presented with such symptoms.[1]

Risk factors

A number of risk factors for ectopic pregnancy have been identified (Table 9.2; see also Chapter 2). It is thought that one-third of all cases of ectopic pregnancy are caused by tubal infection or surgery,[8] with the most common pathogen being *Chlamydia trachomatis*. The majority of women with chlamydial infection are asymptomatic and unaware of previous exposure, and their presentations may vary from cervicitis to florid acute pelvic inflammatory disease. The incidence of tubal damage increases after successive episodes of pelvic inflammatory disease (13% after a single episode, 35% after two episodes and 75% after three episodes).

Another one-third of cases of ectopic pregnancy are thought to be associated with smoking.[8] There is a dose–effect relationship, with the highest adjusted odds ratio (3.9) occurring when more than 20 cigarettes are smoked

TABLE 9.2 **Risk factors for ectopic pregnancy**

Risk factor	Adjusted OR (95% CI)	OR (95% CI)
High risk		
Previous tubal surgery	4.0 (2.6–6.1)	4.7–21.0
Sterilisation		9.3 (4.9–18.0)
Previous ectopic pregnancy		8.3 (6.0–11.5)
Diethylstilbestrol exposure		5.6 (2.4–13.0)
Current use of an IUCD		4.2–45.0
Documented tubal pathology	3.7 (1.2–4.8)	3.8–21.0
Moderate risk		
Infertility	2.1–2.7	2.5–21.0
Previous genital infections		2.5–3.7
Multiple sexual partners		2.1–2.5
Previous termination	2.8 (1.1–7.2)	
Previous miscarriage	3.0 (>2)	
Age >40 years	2.9 (1.4–6.1)	
Slight risk		
Previous pelvic/abdominal surgery		0.9–3.8
Ruptured appendix		1.8 (1.2–2.7)
Cigarette smoking	1.7–3.9	2.3–2.5
Vaginal douching		1.1–3.1
Age <18 years at first intercourse		1.6

Adjusted OR was adjusted for previous pelvic infection, smoking, area, level of education and age. IUCD = intrauterine contraceptive device.

SOURCES: Pisarska M D, Carson S A, Buster J E. Ectopic pregnancy. *Lancet* 1998;351:1115–20 | Farquhar C M. Ectopic pregnancy. *Lancet* 2005;366:583–91 | Bouyer J, Coste J, Shojaci T, Pouly J L, Fernandez H, Gerbaud L, et al. Risk factors for ectopic pregnancy: a comprehensive analysis based on a large case-control, population-based study in France. *Am J Epidemiol* 2003;157:185–94.

each day.[9] Several mechanisms by which cigarette smoking may play a role in ectopic pregnancy have been suggested. These mechanisms include one or more of the following: delayed ovulation, altered tubal and uterine motility and altered immunity.

The risk of ectopic pregnancy is higher in women who have had a previous ectopic pregnancy and increases further in proportion to the number of previous ectopic pregnancies. In one study the odds ratio for having an ectopic pregnancy was 12.5 after one previous ectopic pregnancy and 76.6 after two previous ectopic pregnancies.[9] There is also a significant relationship between advancing age and ectopic pregnancy.[9] Possible explanations for this trend include higher probability of exposure to most risk factors with advancing age and an increase in chromosomal abnormalities and age-related changes in tubal function delaying ovum transport and resulting in tubal implantation.

The use of some types of contraception is associated with an increased risk of ectopic pregnancy. The likelihood of an ectopic pregnancy in women with an intrauterine contraceptive device in place at the time of conception varies from one in two in women with a levonorgestrel-releasing device to one in 16 in women with a copper device.[10] Although progesterone-only contraceptives protect against ectopic pregnancy in general by lowering the chance of conception, if users do get pregnant an average of 6–10% will have an ectopic pregnancy.[11]

Women undergoing in vitro fertilisation have an increased risk of ectopic pregnancy. Studies have shown ectopic pregnancy rates of 4–5% in these women, 2–3% higher than those seen in the general population.[12, 13] The main cause is thought to be retrograde embryo migration into diseased fallopian tubes.[14, 15] Heterotopic pregnancies are also more common (1–3%) following in vitro fertilisation and fertility treatments involving superovulatory drugs.[16, 17]

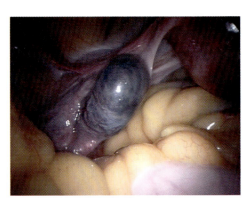

FIGURE 9.1 **Laparoscopic view of an unruptured left ampullary tubal ectopic pregnancy**

Courtesy of Mr Ertan Saridogan, University College Hospital, London.

Surgical diagnosis

Historically, ectopic pregnancies were diagnosed at the time of surgery, and still today some are not diagnosed until the time of laparoscopy or laparotomy. Macroscopically there may be haemoperitoneum with a distended fallopian tube. Microscopically there will be chorionic villi within the tube. There may also be signs of rupture of the tube (Figure 9.1).

Surgical diagnosis is still considered by many as the gold standard for diagnosing an ectopic pregnancy. However, some small ectopic pregnancies can be missed at the time of laparoscopy or laparotomy. In one study, two of 44 (4.5%) women reported to have no evidence of an ectopic pregnancy at the time of laparoscopy were subsequently diagnosed with an ectopic pregnancy.[18] Therefore, if laparoscopy is used routinely as the diagnostic tool for ectopic pregnancy, there is a considerable risk of performing unnecessary operations.

Ultrasound diagnosis

Transvaginal sonography (TVS) has revolutionised the diagnosis of ectopic pregnancy and is now the diagnostic test of choice. Studies have shown that it is an acceptable diagnostic procedure for women presenting with problems such as bleeding and pain in early pregnancy.[19,20]

Criteria for ultrasound diagnosis of tubal ectopic pregnancy

To make a diagnosis of tubal ectopic pregnancy on ultrasound, the aim should be to visualise an ectopic mass rather than just to exclude an intrauterine pregnancy. If neither an intrauterine nor an extrauterine pregnancy is visualised on TVS, the woman should be classified as having a pregnancy of unknown location and then followed up until the final outcome is known.

The following criteria can be used to diagnose a tubal ectopic pregnancy when seen in the adnexa separate to the ovary: an inhomogeneous adnexal mass, an empty extrauterine sac with a hyperechoic ring or a yolk sac and/or fetal pole with or without cardiac activity in an extrauterine sac (Figures 9.2, 9.3 and 9.4). In a meta-analysis of ten studies, the most effective criterion on which to base the diagnosis of ectopic pregnancy was a non-cystic adnexal mass or an inhomogeneous mass. This finding gave a specificity, positive predictive value, sensitivity and negative predictive value of 98.9%, 96.3%, 84.4% and 94.8%, respectively.[21]

A number of other findings may suggest the presence of a tubal ectopic pregnancy, but they are not diagnostic. There may be anechoic or echogenic free fluid within the pelvis. Echogenic fluid within the pouch of Douglas or the pouch of Morrison may suggest haemoperitoneum secondary to a ruptured ectopic pregnancy or a tubal miscarriage, but it may also be seen with rupture of a haemorrhagic ovarian cyst (Figure 9.5). There may also be a collection of fluid within the endometrial cavity, often referred to as a pseudosac (Figure 9.6). Using TVS it is not difficult to distinguish a pseudosac from an early intrauterine gestational sac (Figure 9.7), which is seen as an eccentrically placed hyperechoic ring within the endometrial cavity.

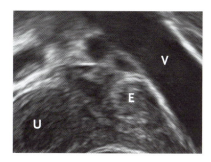

FIGURE 9.2 **Ultrasound scan showing a small left tubal ectopic pregnancy (E), which appeared as a solid, hyperechoic swelling between the uterus (U) and the left external iliac vein (V)**

These findings are typical of a tubal miscarriage.

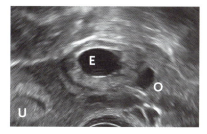

FIGURE 9.3 **Tubal ectopic pregnancy (E) located between the uterus (U) and the left ovary (O)**

The gestational sac is empty with no evidence of a yolk sac or an embryo.

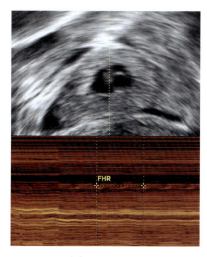

FIGURE 9.4 **Tubal ectopic pregnancy at 8 weeks of gestation containing a live embryo**

Cardiac activity is documented on M-mode.

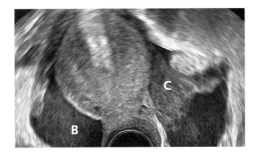

FIGURE 9.5 **Longitudinal section through the uterus showing an empty uterine cavity**

A large amount of echogenic fluid representing blood is seen anterior and posterior to the uterus (B). Blood clots appear as solid, hyperechoic material (C).

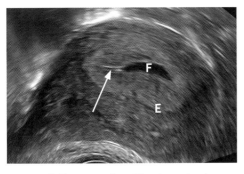

FIGURE 9.6 **Transverse view of the uterus showing a small amount of fluid within the cavity resembling a gestational sac (F).**

By following the midline endometrial echo (arrow), it is possible to establish that the fluid is located between two endometrial layers rather than underneath the endometrial surface. This is the typical appearance of a pseudo-gestational sac. E = endometrium.

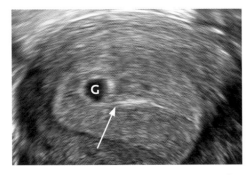

FIGURE 9.7 **Normal intrauterine pregnancy at 4 weeks of gestation**

A gestational sac (G) is embedded below the midline endometrial echo (arrow) and is surrounded by a thick hyperechoic layer of tissue representing trophoblast.

Sensitivity of ultrasound for the diagnosis of ectopic pregnancy

TVS has been shown to have a high sensitivity for the diagnosis of ectopic pregnancy. Studies report sensitivities of 87.0–99.0% with specificities of 94.0–99.9%.[3,22–26] However, the majority of these studies included follow-up ultrasound examinations, so not all of the ectopic pregnancies were detected on the initial examination. Some women would initially have had inconclusive findings and been classified as having a pregnancy of unknown location. Their ectopic pregnancies would then have been visualised on subsequent TVS examinations.

In a prospective study on 5318 women attending an early pregnancy unit over a 1-year period it was found that 91.3% of women had the location of their pregnancy identified on the initial TVS examination.[3] In these women, 89.6% of pregnancies were intrauterine and 1.7% were ectopic, with the remaining 8.7% initially classified as a pregnancy of unknown location. Only 6.8% of the women classified as having a pregnancy of unknown location were subsequently found to have an ectopic pregnancy. The sensitivity of the initial TVS in the diagnosis of ectopic pregnancy was 73.9% with a specificity of 99.9%. However, if follow-up TVS examinations are included, the overall sensitivity of TVS to diagnose an ectopic pregnancy was 98.3% with a specificity of 99.9%. This means that almost 75% of the ectopic pregnancies were visualised on the initial TVS examination, with the remaining 25% arising in women with a pregnancy of unknown location.

There may be a number of reasons why an ectopic pregnancy is not visualised on the initial TVS examination. These include an inexperienced ultrasound operator, poor-quality ultrasound equipment or examination technique, increased body mass index or the presence of pathology such as uterine fibroids or ovarian cysts making visualisation of the adnexa difficult. However, ectopic pregnancy itself may also have features that make it difficult to visualise at the time of the initial TVS examination. A study has compared TVS findings and serum human chorionic gonadotrophin (hCG) levels in women with ectopic pregnancies who had their ectopic pregnancies visualised on the initial TVS examination and in women who were initially classified as having a pregnancy of unknown location.[26] It was found that women who were classified as having a pregnancy of unknown location presented at a significantly earlier mean gestational age and had lower serum hCG levels at the time of the initial assessment compared with women who had their ectopic pregnancies visualised on the initial TVS.[26] However, in a comparison of serum hCG levels at the time of visualisation of the ectopic pregnancy on TVS, there was no significant difference between the two groups, but women initially classified as having a pregnancy of unknown location had significantly smaller ectopic pregnancies. It was concluded that the reason women with ectopic pregnancies who are initially classified as having a pregnancy of unknown location do not have their ectopic pregnancies visualised on the initial TVS is that the pregnancies are too small to be seen and the women present very early in the course of the condition.

Prediction of ectopic pregnancy in women with a pregnancy of unknown location

It is reported that between 7% and 20% of women initially classified as having a pregnancy of unknown location will subsequently be diagnosed with an ectopic pregnancy.[27–30] Expectant management has been shown to be safe for haemodynamically stable women classified as having a pregnancy of unknown location as the majority have a low risk of ectopic pregnancy.[27,29,31] At present there is no consensus on what is an acceptable intervention rate in this group; however, studies report interventions in 0.3–11% of cases.[17,27,30,32] Women with a pregnancy of unknown location are followed up with hormone measurements, repeat TVS examinations and, possibly, laparoscopy or curettage until a diagnosis is confirmed.

Serum hCG
Serum hCG is the most commonly used hormone in the assessment of women in whom ultrasound findings are non-diagnostic. Early studies suggested that a single measurement of serum hCG above a certain level could be used to diagnose an ectopic pregnancy in the absence of an intrauterine pregnancy on ultrasound scan. A cut-off serum hCG of over 6500 iu/l was proposed for use with transabdominal scanning and over 1000–2000 iu/l for use with transvaginal scanning.[28,33] However, it has been shown that using a

single value of serum hCG to predict outcome in women with a pregnancy of unknown location is of limited value. Many ectopic pregnancies will have relatively low serum hCG levels, below the discriminatory zone, so clinicians will be falsely reassured about the location of the pregnancy. In one study, 78% of women with an ectopic pregnancy that was initially classified as a pregnancy of unknown location had an initial serum hCG level below 1000 iu/l.[30] Conversely, some women in the pregnancy of unknown location population who have non-ectopic pregnancies will have very high serum hCG levels, leading to possible inappropriate and unnecessary intervention.

Serial hCG levels are more useful. Many studies have looked at the behaviour of hCG levels in predicting intrauterine pregnancies and pregnancies that are destined to fail. However, the behaviour of serum hCG levels in ectopic pregnancies in women with a pregnancy of unknown location is more difficult to interpret. There is no single way to characterise the behaviour of serum hCG levels in ectopic pregnancies. While the majority of ectopic pregnancies will show a 'suboptimal rise' in hCG over 48 hours (often defined as a rise of less than 66%), 15–20% of ectopic pregnancies will have an hCG profile that mimics a viable intrauterine pregnancy and 8% will have an hCG profile that mimics a spontaneous miscarriage.[34,35]

Serum progesterone

While progesterone levels are good at predicting pregnancy viability, they are relatively poor at predicting pregnancy location. Levels below 20 nmol/l have a high positive predictive value for predicting failing pregnancies,[27] while levels over 25 nmol/l are 'likely to predict' and levels over 60 nmol/l are 'strongly associated with' viable pregnancies.[36] Studies have shown that a single measurement of serum progesterone can identify women at risk of ectopic pregnancy, but its discriminative capacity is insufficient to diagnose ectopic pregnancy with certainty.[37]

Mathematical models

A number of mathematical models have been developed to predict ectopic pregnancy and other possible pregnancy outcomes (intrauterine pregnancy, failing pregnancy of unknown location) in women with a pregnancy of unknown location. Models based on serum hCG levels taken at 0 and 48 hours after presentation have been found to have sensitivities of over 80% for the prediction of ectopic pregnancy.[38,39] When tested in the clinical setting, these models have been shown to compare favourably with subjective assessment by experienced nurse practitioners.[40] A model has also been used to rationalise the follow-up of women with pregnancy of unknown location.[30]

Conclusions

There has been a change in the presentation of tubal ectopic pregnancy over recent years. Fortunately, it is now a relatively rare occurrence to have a woman presenting in a haemodynamically unstable state with an acute abdomen. Surgical diagnosis is no longer the norm. TVS has become the diagnostic modality of choice. More than 90% of ectopic pregnancies can be visualised on TVS prior to treatment. Three-quarters of these pregnancies can be detected on the initial examination. Diagnosis should be based on the positive visualisation of an adnexal mass rather than the inability to visualise an intrauterine pregnancy. The remainder of women will be classified as having a pregnancy of unknown location. These women can then be followed up using a combination of ultrasound and serum hormone levels until a diagnosis of ectopic pregnancy can be made.

References

1 The Confidential Enquiry into Maternal and Child Health (CEMACH). *Saving Mothers' Lives: Reviewing maternal deaths to make motherhood safer – 2003–2005. The Seventh Report of the Confidential Enquiries into Maternal Deaths in the United Kingdom*. London: CEMACH; 2007.

2 Elson J, Tailor A, Banerjee S, Salim R, Hillaby K, Jurkovic D. Expectant management of tubal ectopic pregnancy: prediction of successful outcome using decision tree analysis. *Ultrasound Obstet Gynecol* 2004;23:552–6.

3 Kirk E, Papageorghiou A T, Condous G, Tan L, Bora S, Bourne T. The diagnostic effectiveness of an initial transvaginal scan in detecting ectopic pregnancy. *Hum Reprod* 2007;22:2824–8.

4 Weckstein L N, Boucher A R, Tucker H, Gibson D, Rettenmaier MA. Accurate diagnosis of early ectopic pregnancy. *Obstet Gynecol* 1985;65:393–7.

5 Tay J L, Moore J, Walker J J. Ectopic pregnancy. *BMJ* 2000;320:916–9.

6 Kaplan B C, Dart R G, Moskos M, Kuligowska E, Chun B, Adel Hamid M, et al. Ectopic pregnancy: prospective study with improved diagnostic accuracy. *Ann Emerg Med* 1996;28:10–7.

7 Lewis G, Drife J, editors. *Why Mothers Die 1997–1999. The fifth report of the Confidential Enquiries into Maternal Deaths in the United Kingdom*. London: RCOG Press; 2001.

8 Ankum W M, Mol B W J, Van der Veen F, Bossuyt P M. Risk factors for ectopic pregnancy: a meta analysis. *Fertil Steril* 1996;65:1093–9.

9 Bouyer J, Coste J, Shojaei T, Pouly J L, Fernandez H, Gerbaud L, et al. Risk factors for ectopic pregnancy: a comprehensive analysis based on a large case–control, population-based study in France. *Am J Epidemiol* 2003;157:185–94.

10 Furlong L A. Ectopic pregnancy risk when contraception fails: a review. *J Reprod Med* 2002;47:881–5.

11 McCann M F, Potter L S. Progestin-only oral contraception: a comprehensive review. *Contraception* 1994;50 Suppl 1:S9–S195.

12 Assisted reproductive technology in the United States and Canada: 1992 results generated from the American Fertility Society/Society for Assisted Reproductive Technology Registry. *Fertil Steril* 1994;62:1121–8.

13 Assisted reproductive technology in the United States and Canada: 1994 results generated from the American Fertility Society/Society for Assisted Reproductive Technology Registry. *Fertil Steril* 1996;66:697–705.

14 Nazari A, Askari H A, Check J H, O'Shaughnessy A O. Embryo transfer techniques as a cause of ectopic pregnancy in in vitro fertilization. *Fertil Steril* 1993;60:919–21.

15 Herman A, Ron-El R, Golan A, Weinraub Z, Bukovsky I, Caspi E. The role of tubal pathology and other parameters in ectopic pregnancies occurring in vitro fertilization embryo transfer. *Fetil Steril* 1990;54:864–8.

16 Rojansky N, Schenker J G. Heterotopic pregnancy and assisted reproduction – an update. *J Assist Reprod Genet* 1996;13:594–601.

17 Condous G, Okaro E, Bourne T. The conservative management of early pregnancy complications: a review of the literature. *Ultrasound Obstet Gynecol* 2003;22:420–30.

18 Li T C, Tristram A, Hill A S, Cooke I D. A review of 254 ectopic pregnancies in a teaching hospital in the Trent Region, 1977–1990. *Hum Reprod* 1991;6:1002–7.

19 Dutta R L, Economides D L. Patient acceptance of transvaginal sonography in the early pregnancy unit setting. *Ultrasound Obstet Gynecol* 2003;22:503–7.

20 Basama F M, Crosfill F, Price A. Women's perception of transvaginal sonography in the first trimester; in an early pregnancy assessment unit. *Arch Gynecol Obstet* 2004;269:117–20.

21 Brown D L, Doubilet P M. Transvaginal sonography for diagnosing ectopic pregnancy: positivity criteria and performance characteristics. *J Ultrasound Med* 1994;13:259–66.

22 Braffman B H, Coleman B G, Ramchandani P, Arger P H, Nodine C F, Dinsmore B J, et al. Emergency department screening for ectopic pregnancy: a prospective US study. *Radiology* 1994;190:797–802.

23 Shalev E, Yarom I, Bustan M, Weiner E, Ben-Shlomo I. Transvaginal sonography as the ultimate diagnostic tool for the management of ectopic pregnancy: experience with 840 cases. *Fertil Steril* 1998;69:62–5.

24 Atri M, Valenti D A, Bret P M, Gillett P. Effect of transvaginal sonography on the use of invasive procedures for evaluating patients with a clinical diagnosis of ectopic pregnancy. *J Clin Ultrasound* 2003;31:1–8.

25 Condous G, Okaro E, Khalid A, Lu C, Van Huffel S, Bourne T. The accuracy of transvaginal ultrasonography for the diagnosis of ectopic pregnancy prior to surgery. *Hum Reprod* 2005;20:1404–9.

26 Kirk E, Daemen A, Papageorghiou A T, Bottomley C, Condous G, Moor B D, et al. Why are some ectopic pregnancies characterized as pregnancies of unknown location at the initial transvaginal ultrasound examination? *Acta Obstet Gynecol Scand* 2008;87:1150–4.

27 Banerjee S, Aslam N, Woelfer B, Lawrence A, Elson J, Jurkovic D. Expectant management of early pregnancies of unknown location: a prospective evaluation of methods to predict spontaneous resolution of pregnancy. *BJOG* 2001;108:158–63.

28 Condous G, Kirk E, Lu C, Van Huffel S, Gevaert O, De Moor B, et al. Diagnostic accuracy of varying discriminatory zones for the prediction of ectopic pregnancy in women with a pregnancy of unknown location. *Ultrasound Obstet Gynecol* 2005;26:770–5.

29 Hahlin M, Thorburn J, Bryman I. The expectant management of early pregnancies of uncertain site. *Hum Reprod* 1995;10:1223–7.

30 Kirk E, Condous G, Van Calster B, Van Huffel S, Timmerman D, Bourne T. Rationalizing the follow-up of pregnancies of unknown location. *Hum Reprod* 2007;22:1744–50.

31 Banerjee S, Aslam N, Zosmer N, Woelfer B, Jurkovic D. The expectant management of women with pregnancies of unknown location. *Ultrasound Obstet Gynecol* 1999;14: 231–6.

32 Condous G, Timmerman D, Goldstein S, Valentin L, Jurkovic D, Bourne T. Pregnancies of unknown location: consensus statement. *Ultrasound Obstet Gynecol* 2006;28:121–2.

33 Romero R, Kadar N, Jeanty P, Copel J A, Chervenak F A, DeCherney A, et al. Diagnosis of ectopic pregnancy: value of the discriminatory human chorionic gonadotropin zone. *Obstet Gynecol* 1985;66:357–60.

34 Silva C, Sammel M D, Zhou L, Gracia C, Hummel A C, Barnhart K. Human chorionic gonadotrophin profile for women with ectopic pregnancy. *Obstet Gynecol* 2006; 107:605–10.

35 Goldstein S. The diagnosis of miscarriage. In: Bourne T H, Coundous G, editors. *Handbook of Early Pregnancy Care.* London: Informa Healthcare; 2006. p. 27–35.

36 Royal College of Obstetricians and Gynaecologists. Green-top Guideline No. 25. *The management of early pregnancy loss*. London; RCOG: 2006 [www.rcog.org.uk/files/womens-health/clinical-guidance/management-early-pregnancy-loss-green-top-25].

37 Mol B W, Lijmer J G, Ankum W, van der Veen F, Bossuyt P M. The accuracy of single serum progesterone measurement in the diagnosis of ectopic pregnancy: a meta-analysis. *Hum Reprod* 1998;13:3220–7.

38 Condous G, Okaro E, Khalid A, Timmerman D, Lu C, Zhou Y, et al. The use of a new logistic regression model for predicting the outcome of pregnancies of unknown location. *Hum Reprod* 2004;19:1900–10.

39 Condous G, Van Calster B, Kirk E, Haider Z, Timmerman D, Van Huffel S, et al. Prediction of ectopic pregnancy in women with a pregnancy of unknown location. *Ultrasound Obstet Gynecol* 2007;29:680–7.

40 Kirk E, Condous G, Haider Z, Lu C, Van Huffel S, Timmerman D, et al. The practical application of a mathematical model to predict the outcome of pregnancies of unknown location. *Ultrasound Obstet Gynecol* 2006;27:311–15.

10 Conservative management of tubal ectopic pregnancy

Petra J Hajenius and Norah M van Mello

Introduction

Recent advances in ultrasound diagnosis and the high sensitivity of modern urinary pregnancy tests have enabled the diagnosis of many cases of small tubal ectopic pregnancies that were undetectable in the past. Many of these pregnancies represent early tubal ectopic pregnancies or tubal miscarriages that are eligible for non-surgical treatment, such as medical treatment and expectant management.

Medical treatment is mainly focused on systemic methotrexate, which is the most commonly used drug in clinical practice. Methotrexate facilitates non-invasive outpatient management of ectopic pregnancy. Systemic methotrexate and expectant management are used only in women with a low risk of complications, such as a small ectopic pregnancy, low serum human chorionic gonadotrophin (hCG) concentration and no signs of intra-abdominal bleeding. However, these women remain at risk of tubal rupture. Serum hCG monitoring is therefore mandatory to detect impending treatment failure and inadequately declining serum hCG concentrations. Additional methotrexate injections or surgical intervention may then be needed.

This chapter provides an overview of the best available evidence on the conservative management of tubal ectopic pregnancy, both medical treatment with systemic methotrexate and expectant management.

Systemic methotrexate

Methotrexate is a folic acid antagonist that inhibits de novo synthesis of purines and pyrimidines, thereby interfering with DNA synthesis and cell proliferation. Secondary to its effect on highly proliferative tissues such as trophoblast, methotrexate has a strong dose-related potential for toxicity. Adverse effects of systemic methotrexate include stomatitis, conjunctivitis, gastritis–enteritis, impaired liver function, bone marrow depression and photosensitivity.[1]

TABLE 10.1 **Evidence on medical treatment with methotrexate for tubal ectopic pregnancy**

First author, year of publication, country	Patients	Intervention	Comparison	Treatment success RR (95% CI)	Quality features
Systemic methotrexate in a fixed multiple-dose regimen versus laparoscopic salpingotomy					
Hajenius et al., 1997 The Netherlands	$n=100$; laparoscopically confirmed; no fetal cardiac activity; no limit on EP size; no upper limit for serum hCG	Multiple-dose MTX (1.0 mg/kg IM on days 0, 2, 4 and 6 alternated with folinic acid 0.1 mg/kg orally on days 1, 3, 5 and 7)	Laparoscopic salpingotomy	1.2 (0.93–1.4)	Block randomisation by a computer program; allocation adequate; power calculation performed; intention-to-treat analysis; multicentre
Systemic methotrexate in a single-dose regimen versus laparoscopic salpingotomy					
El-Sherbiny et al., 2003 Egypt	$n=55$; EP <4 cm; no fetal cardiac activity; serum hCG < 10 000 iu/l	Single-dose MTX (50 mg/m^2 IM)	Laparoscopic salpingotomy	0.79 (0.59–1.1)	Randomisation by computer; allocation unclear; no power calculation; multicentre
Fernandez et al., 1998 France	$n=100$; EP confirmed by TVS/TAS; pretherapeutic score <13; size NR; fetal cardiac activity NR; upper limit for serum hCG NR	Single-dose MTX (1 mg/kg IM)	Laparoscopic salpingotomy	0.71 (0.53–0.95)	Randomisation using a random number table; allocation unclear; no power calculation; single centre
Saraj et al., 1998 USA	$n=75$; EP <3.5 cm on TVS; no fetal cardiac activity; upper limit for serum hCG NR	Single-dose MTX (1 mg/kg IM)	Laparoscopic salpingotomy	0.86 (0.71–1.0)	Randomisation NR; allocation unclear, although sealed envelopes; no power calculation; multicentre
Sowter et al., 2001 New Zealand	$n=62$; EP <3.5 cm; no fetal cardiac activity; serum hCG <5000 iu/l	Single-dose MTX (50 mg/m^2 IM)	Laparoscopic salpingotomy	0.95 (0.67–1.4)	Unblocked randomisation procedure by a computer program; allocation by envelopes sealed by a third party; power calculation performed; intention-to-treat analysis; multicentre
				Combined result: 0.82 (0.72–0.94)	

continued

First author, year of publication, country	Patients	Intervention	Comparison	Treatment success RR (95% CI)	Quality features
Single-dose versus multiple-dose systemic methotrexate					
Klauser et al., 2005 USA	$n = 51$; serum hCG <10 000 iu/l; size NR; fetal cardiac activity NR	Single-dose MTX (50 mg/m^2 IM)	Multiple-dose MTX (1 mg/kg IM on days 1, 3 and 5)	1.05 (0.87–1.3)	Randomisation NR; allocation unclear; no power calculation; single centre
Alleyassin et al., 2006 Iran	$n = 108$; EP <3.5 cm on TVS; no fetal cardiac activity; serum hCG <15 000 iu/l	Single-dose MTX (50 mg/m^2 IM)	Multiple-dose MTX (1.0 mg/kg IM on days 0, 2, 4 and 6 alternated with folinic acid 0.1 mg/kg orally on days 1, 3, 5 and 7)	0.96 (0.85–1.1)	Block randomisation by computer-generated random table; allocation by sealed envelopes; no blinding; power calculation performed; single centre
				Combined result: 0.99 (0.89–1.1)	
Systemic methotrexate in different dosages					
Yalcinkaya et al., 2000 USA	$n = 100$; EP <3.5 cm on TVS; fetal cardiac activity allowed; rising/plateauing hCG; upper limit for serum hCG NR	Single-dose MTX (25 mg/m^2 IM)	Single-dose MTX (50 mg/m^2 IM)	0.87 (0.65–1.2)	Randomisation method NR; allocation adequate by sealed envelopes at central pharmacy; double-blind; single centre; power calculation performed
Systemic methotrexate alone versus systemic methotrexate in combination with mifepristone					
Gazvani et al., 1998 UK	$n = 50$; EP <4 cm on TVS; laparoscopically confirmed unruptured tubal pregnancy	Single-dose systemic MTX (50 mg/m^2 IM)	Single-dose systemic MTX (50 mg/m^2 IM) in combination with mifepristone 600 mg orally	0.82 (0.62–1.1)	Randomisation by computer-generated random table; consecutively numbered envelopes; no power calculation; single centre; intention-to-treat analysis
Rozenberg et al., 2003 France	$n = 212$; EP confirmed by algorithm combining TVS, serum hCG and/or curettage showing no trophoblastic villi	Single-dose systemic MTX (50 mg/m^2 IM)	Single-dose systemic MTX (50 mg/m^2 IM) in combination with mifepristone 600 mg orally	0.85 (0.69–1.0)	Block randomisation by computer; sealed envelopes; double-blind, placebo-controlled study; multicentre; power calculation was performed; intention-to-treat analysis
				Combined result: 0.84 (0.71–1.0)	

EP = ectopic pregnancy | hCG = human chorionic gonadotrophin | IM = intramuscularly | MTX = methotrexate |
NR = not registered | TAS = transabdominal ultrasound | TVS = transvaginal ultrasound.

Systemic methotrexate can be given intramuscularly in a fixed multiple-dose regimen or in a single-dose regimen. The fixed multiple-dose regimen comprises a total of four injections of methotrexate 1 mg/kg intramuscularly alternating with folinic acid (citrovorum/leucovorin rescue) 0.1 mg/kg intramuscularly or orally 24 hours after each methotrexate injection to reduce drug toxicity.[2] The single-dose regimen was introduced to improve compliance, minimise adverse effects and reduce overall costs. In clinical practice, additional methotrexate injections for inadequately declining serum hCG concentrations are frequently necessary, resulting in an individualised variable-dose regimen comprising single methotrexate injections without folinic acid rescue.

Serum hCG clearance curves after systemic methotrexate treatment can be used by clinicians to monitor the success of treatment and to detect potential treatment failures.[3–6]

We assessed ten randomised controlled trials of systemic methotrexate for the treatment of tubal pregnancy (Table 10.1), focusing on five clinically relevant comparisons:

- systemic methotrexate in a fixed multiple-dose regimen versus laparoscopic salpingotomy (one trial)

- systemic methotrexate in a single-dose regimen versus laparoscopic salpingotomy (four trials)

- single-dose versus multiple-dose systemic methotrexate (two trials)

- systemic methotrexate in different doses (one trial)

- systemic methotrexate alone versus systemic methotrexate in combination with mifepristone (two trials).

Systemic methotrexate in a fixed multiple-dose regimen compared with laparoscopic salpingotomy

In a multicentre trial, 100 haemodynamically stable women with a laparoscopically confirmed unruptured tubal ectopic pregnancy without fetal cardiac activity and no signs of active intra-abdominal bleeding were randomly allocated to either systemic methotrexate in a fixed multiple dose (methotrexate 1 mg/kg intramuscularly on days 0, 2, 4 and 6 alternated with folinic acid 0.1 mg/kg orally on days 1, 3, 5 and 7) or laparoscopic salpingotomy.[4] A second course was given on day 14 if the serum hCG concentration on that day was more than 40% above the initial value on day 0. There were no limits on serum hCG concentration or size of the ectopic pregnancy. The mean serum hCG concentration in women treated with systemic methotrexate was 1950 iu/l (range 110–19 500 iu/l). There was a non-significant trend towards a higher rate of treatment success with systemic methotrexate treatment (RR 1.2, 95% CI 0.93–1.4).

In a scenario analysis it was calculated that systemic methotrexate, if administered as part of a non-invasive treatment strategy, was less costly only in women with initial serum hCG concentrations below 1500 iu/l, equally costly if the initial serum hCG concentration ranged between 1500 iu/l and 3000 iu/l and more costly in women with initial serum hCG concentrations over 3000 iu/l compared with laparoscopic surgery.[7] Health-related quality of life was impaired to a greater extent after systemic methotrexate.[8] However, in a case–control study women indicated that they were willing to trade off the increased treatment burden of systemic methotrexate for the benefit of non-invasive management of tubal ectopic pregnancy.[9]

Systemic methotrexate in a single-dose regimen compared with laparoscopic salpingotomy

The combined results of four trials involving a total of 265 haemodynamically stable women with a small unruptured tubal ectopic pregnancy showed that single-dose systemic methotrexate (50 mg/m² or 1 mg/kg intramuscularly) was significantly less successful than laparoscopic salpingotomy (RR 0.82, 95% CI 0.72–0.94).[6,10–12] The selection criteria used in these trials were an upper limit of serum hCG below 5000–10 000 iu/l, absence of positive fetal heartbeat and small size of the ectopic pregnancy (under 3.5–4 cm). The mean serum hCG concentrations in women treated with systemic methotrexate varied between 927 and 3162 iu/l.

Additional injections for inadequately declining serum hCG concentrations were frequently necessary, eventually resulting in a variable-dose methotrexate regimen. The variable dose regimen comprised a single dose of methotrexate with an additional methotrexate injection if the serum hCG concentration between days 4 and 7 failed to decline by at least 15% of the initial value on day 1. If during any successive week of follow-up serum hCG again failed to fall by at least 15%, a repeat injection of methotrexate was administered. The cumulative treatment success rates after one, two, three or four single doses were 77%, 92%, 93% and 94%, respectively. With this variable-dose regimen, the overall treatment success rate increased, but there was no evidence of a difference compared with laparoscopic salpingotomy (RR 1.0, 95% CI 0.92–1.1).

Systemic methotrexate resulted in significant savings in direct costs compared with laparoscopic surgery.[13] These savings resulted from both reduced theatre usage and shorter hospital stay. Furthermore, systemic methotrexate resulted in a significant saving in indirect costs. However, subgroup analysis showed that cost savings are lost in women with an initial serum hCG concentration over 1,500 iu/l. Women treated with systemic methotrexate had significantly better physical functioning than women who received laparoscopic surgery. No differences were found in psychological functioning between the two groups.[12]

Single-dose compared with multiple-dose systemic methotrexate

The results of two trials comparing the single-dose (50 mg/m²) versus the fixed multiple-dose (1 mg/kg day on days 1, 3 and 5) methotrexate regimen, involving 159 women, showed no significant difference in treatment success rates (RR 0.99, 95% CI 0.89–1.1).[14,15] In the study by Klauser et al. the mean serum hCG concentrations varied between 2230 iu/l and 2973 iu/l in the single-dose group and between 2180 iu/l and 2244 iu/l in the multiple-dose group. The minor adverse effect rate was 28% in the single-dose group compared with 10% in the multiple-dose group.[14] This was in contrast to the findings of Alleyassin et al., who reported adverse effects in 28% of women in the single-dose group compared with 37% in the multiple-dose group.[15] Serum hCG levels in that study were 3146 ± 2389 iu/l in the single-dose group versus 2803 ± 2100 iu/l in the multiple-dose group.

Systemic methotrexate in different doses

A double-blind study involving 100 haemodynamically stable women with an unruptured tubal ectopic pregnancy showed a non-significant tendency towards lower treatment success with a lower dose of methotrexate (25 mg/m²) compared with the standard 50 mg/m² dose (RR 0.87, 95% CI 0.65–1.2).[16] A second methotrexate injection for inadequately declining serum hCG concentrations was necessary in 15 of 48 (31%) women in the lower-dose group and in 13 of 52 (25%) women in the standard group. Treatment success rates did not differ between the two groups. The mean serum hCG concentrations were 2405 ± 3204 iu/l and 2841 ± 4132 iu/l in the lower-dose group and the standard group, respectively, and fetal heart activity was present in two (4.2%) and seven (13.4%) women, respectively.

Systemic methotrexate alone compared with systemic methotrexate in combination with mifepristone

There are two trials comparing systemic methotrexate alone with systemic methotrexate in combination with mifepristone, involving a total of 262 haemodynamically stable women with an unruptured ectopic pregnancy and no signs of intra-abdominal bleeding. Both trials showed that single-dose methotrexate alone (50 mg/m^2) was less successful than the same dose in combination with 600 mg mifepristone (an antiprogesterone) (RR 0.84, 95% CI 0.71–1.0). Although the diagnosis of tubal ectopic pregnancy was confirmed laparoscopically in the first study, the mean serum hCG concentrations were low in both treatment groups: 346 iu/l (range 52–12 700 iu/l) in the methotrexate alone group and 497 iu/l (range 30–4200 iu/l) in the combination treatment group.[17] In the second study, a non-laparoscopic diagnostic algorithm was used to confirm ectopic pregnancy. The mean serum hCG concentrations were 1,679 iu/l (range 652–3658 iu/l) in the methotrexate alone group and 1620 iu/l (range 805–3190 iu/l) in the combination treatment group.[18]

The results of these randomised controlled trials show that systemic methotrexate in a fixed multiple-dose regimen can be used for the treatment of women who are haemodynamically stable with an unruptured tubal ectopic pregnancy and no signs of active intra-abdominal bleeding who present with serum hCG concentrations below 3000 iu/l. In women with serum hCG concentrations below 1500 iu/l, a single-dose methotrexate regimen can be considered. The addition of mifepristone to systemic methotrexate may slightly increase the success rate. Future research should focus on dosage schemes of systemic methotrexate, including adverse effects, women's quality of life and costs.

Expectant management

Expectant management of ectopic pregnancy has been advocated based on the knowledge that the natural course of many early ectopic pregnancies is a self-limiting process, ultimately resulting in tubal miscarriage or reabsorption.[19] Case series have been published describing expectant management in selected women. Success rates in these case series vary between 42% and 100%.[20] Serum hCG dynamics during spontaneous resolution of ectopic pregnancy have been published; however, to date there are no clear criteria for therapeutic intervention.[21]

Two randomised controlled trials have been published on expectant management for ectopic pregnancy (Table 10.2), one comparing expectant management with local and systemic prostaglandins[22] and the other comparing expectant management with systemic methotrexate.[23]

Expectant management compared with local and systemic prostaglandins

One trial compared expectant management with local and systemic prostaglandins in 23 women with an unruptured ectopic pregnancy and a serum hCG concentration below 2500 iu/l.[22] Expectant management was significantly less successful than prostaglandin therapy (RR 0.12, 95% CI 0.02–0.81). This trial was stopped prematurely after the first intermediate analysis because the primary treatment success rate was significantly lower in the expectant management group.

Expectant management compared with systemic methotrexate

In a double-blind, placebo-controlled trial, expectant management was compared with oral low-dosage methotrexate (2.5 mg/day for 5 days) in 60 women who were haemodynamically stable with a small tubal ectopic pregnancy (under 4 cm) without fetal cardiac activity and a serum hCG concentration under 5000 iu/l.[23] This study virtually represents a comparison between two placebo treatments, as demonstrated by the similar success rates of 77% in both treatment groups (RR 1.0, 95% CI 0.76–1.3). The mean serum hCG concentrations were low: 211 iu/l (range 20–1343 iu/l) in the expectant management group and 395 iu/l (range 61–4279 iu/l) in the methotrexate group. This trial is not informative from a clinical viewpoint, as the oral route of administration and the low dosage of methotrexate used are uncommon and likely to fail.

With the results of only two randomised trials available, it is not possible to reach a conclusion about the effectiveness of expectant management of tubal ectopic pregnancy. Two continuing randomised controlled trials are evaluating the expectant management of ectopic pregnancy. The first trial is comparing expectant management versus single-dose systemic methotrexate in women with an ultrasound diagnosis of tubal ectopic pregnancy and a serum hCG concentration below 1500 iu/l.[24] The second trial is comparing expectant management versus single-dose systemic methotrexate in women with an ultrasound diagnosis of tubal ectopic pregnancy and a persistent pregnancy of unknown location (upper limit serum hCG concentration 2000 iu/l).[25]

TABLE 10.2 **Evidence on expectant management for tubal ectopic pregnancy**

First author, year of publication, country	Patients	Intervention	Comparison	Treatment success RR (95% CI)	Quality features
Egarter et al., 1991 Austria	$n=23$; laparoscopically confirmed; serum hCG <2500 iu/l	1.5–2 ml isotonic NaCl solution injected into the tubal pregnancy under laparoscopic guidance versus no medical therapy at all	10 mg PGF2α in 1.5–2 ml into the tubal pregnancy +25 mg conjugated estrogens injected into the ipsilateral ovary under laparoscopic guidance +500 mg synthetic PGE2 derivative IM twice daily during the first 3 postoperative days	0.12 (0.02–0.81)	Randomisation method during laparoscopy NR; interim analysis; power calculation performed
Korhonen et al., 1996 Finland	$n=60$; ectopic pregnancy <4 cm; fetal cardiac activity NR; serum hCG <5000 iu/l	Expectant management	MTX 2.5 mg/day orally for 5 days	1.0 (0.76–1.3)	Randomisation by table of random numbers; allocation adequate by hospital pharmacy; double-blind, placebo-controlled; power calculation performed; single centre

EP = ectopic pregnancy | hCG = human chorionic gonadotrophin | IM = intramuscularly | MTX = methotrexate | PGE = prostaglandin | PGF2α = prostaglandin F2 alpha | NR = not registered | TAS = transabdominal sonography | TVS = transvaginal sonography.

Recommendations for clinical practice

When considering conservative treatment for tubal ectopic pregnancy, women should be given detailed information about the success rate and risk of complications (Table 10.3).[26]

Anti-D prophylaxis should be given to all rhesus-negative women. Follow-up with measurements of serum hCG concentrations is mandatory until the levels become undetectable. A serum hCG clearance curve after multiple-dose systemic methotrexate treatment is shown in Figure 10.1.[4] It is advis-

TABLE 10.3 **Recommendations for clinical practice for conservative management for tubal ectopic pregnancy** [26]

Expectant management	Additional instructions for systemic methotrexate
Pretreatment testing	
Serum hCG concentration	Liver and renal function tests and complete blood count to detect contraindications
Blood type and screening	
Lifestyle	
Adequate patient compliance	Avoidance of gas-forming foods
Refrain from sexual intercourse	Avoidance of alcohol, aspirin, NSAIDs and folic acid supplements
	Avoidance of exposure to sunlight
	Fluid intake of at least 1.5 litres daily
	Daily use of 0.9% saline mouthwashes; in cases of stomatitis, daily use of chlorhexidine 0.12% mouthwashes
Follow-up	
375 IE anti-D IM if rhesus-negative	Complete blood count and liver and renal function tests to detect adverse effects
Serum hCG monitoring until level is undetectable	
Transvaginal sonography	Delay of pregnancy for at least 3 months after treatment owing to the small risk of teratogenicity
Pain relief with paracetamol	

hCG = human chorionic gonadotrophin | IM = intramuscularly | NSAID = non-steroidal anti-inflammatory drug.

able for women to refrain from sexual intercourse during the follow-up period. Paracetamol can be given for pain relief.

Contraindications to systemic methotrexate are evidence of immunodeficiency, moderate to severe anaemia, leucopenia or thrombocytopenia, active peptic ulcer disease and hepatic or renal dysfunction. Prior to the administration of systemic methotrexate women should have a full blood count and undergo liver and renal function tests. These tests can be repeated during follow-up. Women must be informed about the need to comply with the follow-up, abstain from alcohol use and avoid aspirin, non-steroidal anti-inflammatory drugs and fol(in)ic acid supplements. They should also avoid exposure to sunlight and gas-forming foods. Fluid intake should be at least 1.5 litres/day. Women should use 0.9% saline mouthwashes or chlorhexidine 0.12% in cases of stomatitis. Future pregnancies should be delayed for at least 3 months after completion of medical treatment with systemic methotrexate because of the small risk of teratogenicity.

FIGURE 10.1 **Serum human chorionic gonadotrophin clearance curve after multiple-dose systemic methotrexate (MTX)** [4]

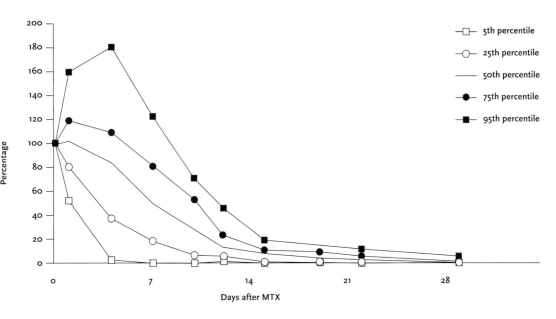

When expectant management is used, no other investigations are required apart from blood type and screening and haemoglobin level.

Conclusion

In conclusion, in selected patients, medical treatment with systemic methotrexate is an alternative non-surgical treatment option for tubal ectopic pregnancy. It is not yet possible to make an adequate evaluation of expectant management of tubal ectopic pregnancy.

References

1 Barnhart K, Coutifaris C, Esposito M. The pharmacology of methotrexate. *Expert Opin Pharmacother* 2001;2:409–17.

2 Hajenius PJ, Mol F, Mol BW, Bossuyt PM, Ankum WM, Van der Veen F. Interventions for tubal ectopic pregnancy. *Cochrane Database Syst Rev* 2007;(1):CD000324.

3 Fernandez H, Bourget P, Ville Y, Lelaidier C, Frydman R. Treatment of unruptured tubal pregnancy with methotrexate: pharmacokinetic analysis of local versus intramuscular administration. *Fertil Steril* 1994;62:943–7.

4 Hajenius PJ, Engelsbel S, Mol BW, Van der Veen F, Ankum WM, Bossuyt-PM, et al. Randomised trial of systemic methotrexate versus laparoscopic salpingostomy in tubal pregnancy. *Lancet* 1997;350:774–9.

5 Natale A, Candiani M, Barbieri M, Calia C, Odorizzi M P, Busacca M. Pre- and post-treatment patterns of human chorionic gonadotropin for early detection of persistence after a single dose of methotrexate for ectopic pregnancy. *Eur J Obstet Gynecol Reprod Biol* 2004;117:87–92.

6 Saraj A J, Wilcox J G, Najmabadi S, Stein S M, Johnson M B, Paulson R J. Resolution of hormonal markers of ectopic gestation: a randomised trial comparing single-dose intramuscular methotrexate with salpingostomy. *Obstet Gynecol* 1998;92:989–94.

7 Mol B W, Hajenius P J, Engelsbel S, Ankum W M, Hemrika D J, Van der Veen F, et al. Treatment of tubal pregnancy in The Netherlands: an economic comparison of systemic methotrexate administration and laparoscopic salpingostomy. *Am J Obstet Gynecol* 1999;181:945–51.

8 Nieuwkerk P T, Hajenius P J, Ankum W M, Van der Veen F, Wijker W, Bossuyt PM. Systemic methotrexate therapy versus laparoscopic salpingostomy in patients with tubal pregnancy. Part I. Impact on patients' health-related quality of life. *Fertil Steril* 1998;70:511–17.

9 Nieuwkerk P T, Hajenius P J, Van der Veen F, Ankum W M, Wijker W, Bossuyt P M. Systemic methotrexate therapy versus laparoscopic salpingostomy in tubal pregnancy. Part II Patient preferences for systemic methotrexate. *Fertil Steril* 1998;7:518–22.

10 El-Sherbiny M T, El G I, Mera I M. Methotrexate versus laparoscopic surgery for the management of unruptured tubal pregnancy. *Middle East Fertility Society Journal* 2003;8:256–62.

11 Fernandez H, Yves Vincent S C, Pauthier S, Audibert F, Frydman R. Randomized trial of conservative laparoscopic treatment and methotrexate administration in ectopic pregnancy and subsequent fertility. *Hum Reprod* 1998;13:3239–43.

12 Sowter M C, Farquhar C M, Petrie K J, Gudex G. A randomised trial comparing single dose systemic methotrexate and laparoscopic surgery for the treatment of unruptured ectopic pregnancy. *BJOG* 2001;108:192–203.

13 Sowter M C, Farquhar C M, Gudex G. An economic evaluation of single dose systemic methotrexate and laparoscopic surgery for the treatment of unruptured ectopic pregnancy. *BJOG* 2001;108:204–12.

14 Klauser C K, May W L, Johnson V K, Cowan B D, Hines R S. Methotrexate for ectopic pregnancy: a randomised single dose compared with multiple dose. *Obstet Gynecol* 2005;105:64S.

15 Alleyassin A, Khademi A, Aghahosseini M, Safdarian L, Badenoosh B, Hamed E A. Comparison of success rates in the medical management of ectopic pregnancy with single-dose and multiple-dose administration of methotrexate: a prospective, randomized clinical trial. *Fertil Steril* 2006;85:1661–6.

16 Yalcinkaya T M, Brown S E, Mertz H L, Thomas D W. A comparison of 25 mg/m2 vs 50 mg/m2 dose of methotrexate (MTX) for the treatment of ectopic pregnancy (EP). *J Soc Gynecol Investig* 2000;7:179A.

17 Gazvani M R, Baruah D N, Alfirevic Z, Emery S J. Mifepristone in combination with methotrexate for the medical treatment of tubal pregnancy: a randomized, controlled trial. *Hum Reprod* 1998;13:1987–90.

18 Rozenberg P, Chevret S, Camus E, de Tayrac R, Garbin O, Poncheville LL, et al. Medical treatment of ectopic pregnancies: a randomized clinical trial comparing methotrexate–mifepristone and methotrexate–placebo. *Hum Reprod* 2003;18:1802–8.

19 Mashiach S, Carp H J, Serr D M. Nonoperative management of ectopic pregnancy. A preliminary report. *J Reprod Med* 1982;27:127–32.

20 Hajenius P J. *Methotrexate in ectopic pregnancy*. Academic thesis, University of Amsterdam, 1998.

21 Korhonen J, Stenman U H, Ylöstalo P. Serum human chorionic gonadotropin dynamics during spontaneous resolution of ectopic pregnancy. *Fertil Steril* 1994;61:632–6.

22 Egarter C, Kiss H, Husslein P. Prostaglandin versus expectant management in early tubal pregnancy. *Prostaglandins Leukot Essent Fatty Acids* 1991;42:177–9.

23 Korhonen J, Stenman U, Ylöstalo P. Low-dose oral methotrexate with expectant management of ectopic pregnancy. *Obstet Gynecol* 1996;88:775–8.

24 Randomised double blind controlled trial of single dose methotrexate versus expectant management in women with tubal ectopic pregnancy [www.controlled-trials.com/ISRCTN95698259/95698259].

25 van Mello N M, Mol F, Adriaanse A H, Boss E A, Dijkman AB, Doornbos JP, et al. The METEX study: methotrexate versus expectant management in women with ectopic pregnancy: a randomised controlled trial. *BMC Womens Health* 2008;8:10.

26 Practice Committee of the American Society for Reproductive Medicine. Medical treatment of ectopic pregnancy. *Fertil Steril* 2006;86 Suppl 1:96–102.

11 Surgical management of tubal ectopic pregnancy

Willem M Ankum, Femke Mol and Amna Jamil

Introduction

Tubal ectopic pregnancies have historically been treated by laparotomy, with removal of the affected tube considered the definitive treatment. This remains the preferred option in cases complicated by major intraperitoneal bleeding and haemorrhagic shock. However, owing to the wide availability of transvaginal ultrasound and sensitive urine pregnancy tests, nowadays most tubal ectopic pregnancies are diagnosed in women who are haemodynamically stable with minimal clinical symptoms. This has led to the introduction of less invasive options for the surgical treatment of tubal ectopic pregnancies. This chapter reviews current strategies for surgical treatment of tubal ectopic pregnancy, focusing on the advantages and disadvantages of the various approaches.

Indications for surgical treatment of tubal ectopic pregnancy

Laparoscopic surgery has evolved from being a main diagnostic to a primary treatment modality as a result of the improved accuracy of non-invasive diagnosis of tubal ectopic pregnancy. In women with a confirmed diagnosis of tubal ectopic pregnancy, the following are the indications for surgical treatment:

- woman who is haemodynamically unstable or evidence of significant intraperitoneal bleeding on ultrasound

- viable tubal ectopic pregnancy

- significant clinical symptoms

- initial serum human chorionic gonadotrophin (hCG) over 3000 iu/ml

- failure of or non-compliance with medical or expectant management

- heterotopic pregnancy with a normal viable intrauterine gestation.

Surgery should not be delayed in women with suspected tubal pregnancy showing signs of hypovolaemic shock. Transvaginal sonography can confirm intra-abdominal bleeding in women with an uncertain diagnosis; however, timely surgical intervention for haemostasis is crucial for resuscitation in those with significant intraperitoneal bleeding.

Surgical approach

Laparoscopy has become the surgical method of choice in haemodynamically stable women with tubal ectopic pregnancy. However, not all tubal ectopic pregnancies are suitable for laparoscopic treatment. The relative contraindications for laparoscopy in tubal pregnancy include evidence of haemodynamic compromise where rapid haemostasis is required, severe pelvic adhesions and insufficient operator experience of laparoscopic surgery.

There is a limited role for laparoscopy in women with a ruptured tubal ectopic pregnancy who show signs of hypovolaemic shock. An experienced laparoscopic surgeon may be able to achieve haemostasis effectively in a short time even in women with a significant haemoperitoneum; however, laparotomy is considered safer for rapid control of bleeding.

Laparoscopic compared with open surgery

Two studies have compared the laparoscopic and open surgical approaches for performing salpingotomy in women with tubal ectopic pregnancies.[1,2] Pooled results from these trials, in a total of 165 women who were haemodynamically stable with small unruptured tubal pregnancies, showed laparoscopic salpingotomy to be significantly less successful than the open surgical approach in terms of elimination of the tubal ectopic pregnancy (RR 0.90, 95% CI 0.82–0.99).[3] The lack of tactile information in laparoscopic salpingotomy could explain the higher rate of persistent trophoblast in comparison with open surgery.

Despite this apparent drawback of laparoscopic surgery, costs were reduced in comparison with the open approach. One of the studies reported savings per woman of €1110, a difference that mainly resulted from the shorter hospital stay after laparoscopy in comparison with open surgery: 1.4 days compared with 3.3 days ($P < 0.001$).[1] The other study showed similar results, with reduced costs for laparoscopic surgery in comparison with open surgery (€2986 compared with €3480, $P = 0.03$), mainly as a result of a shorter operation time (73 minutes compared with 88 minutes, $P < 0.001$), less blood loss (79 ml against

195 ml, $P < 0.01$), a shorter hospital stay (2 days compared with 5 days, $P < 0.01$) and a quicker recovery time (11 days against 24 days, $P < 0.001$).[2,4]

Long-term follow-up was assessed in 127 women.[5,6] The number of subsequent intrauterine pregnancies did not differ (RR 1.08, 95% CI 0.80–1.48), while a non-significant tendency towards a lower repeat tubal ectopic pregnancy rate after laparoscopic surgery was found (RR 0.48, 95% CI 0.16–1.49).

No randomised data comparing laparoscopic with open salpingectomy are available. Since persistent trophoblast is extremely rare after salpingectomy, it seems clear that the results of such a hypothetical trial would favour the laparoscopic approach.

Linear salpingostomy compared with salpingectomy

Linear salpingostomy

Linear salpingostomy involves removal of products of conception with preservation of the affected tube. Diluted vasopressin (0.2 iu/ml) can be injected into the area of maximum distension in the tube. A longitudinal incision is made in the antimesosalpingeal border of the tube with unipolar needle electrocautery or scissors. The gestational products are then flushed out with hydrodissection using a suction irrigator. The tubal stoma is left open to heal with secondary intention. There is no difference in tubal patency rates and subsequent intrauterine pregnancies with or without suturing of the opening.[7,8] All women who have undergone a linear salpingostomy should routinely be followed up with weekly hCG, as there is a 5–20% risk of residual trophoblastic tissue.

Salpingectomy

Salpingectomy is the partial or complete removal of the fallopian tube containing the tubal ectopic pregnancy. Indications for salpingectomy include:

- evidence of tubal rupture or severe tubal damage

- recurrence of ectopic pregnancy in the same tube

- non-availability of surgical expertise for conservative surgical treatment

- inability to achieve haemostasis after salpingostomy

- no desire for future fertility.

The surgical approach to open salpingectomy usually involves a Pfannenstiel or low vertical midline incision. The affected tube is mobilised and elevated and the mesosalpinx is clamped as close to the fallopian tube as possible. The entire length of the fallopian tube is then excised. A small myometrial wedge is cut at the level of the uterine insertion of the tube and the defect is closed with a figure-of-eight mattress suture. The mesosalpinx is sutured with interrupted ligatures.

The surgical technique at laparoscopic salpingectomy is similar and involves the use of endoscopic stapling devices, bipolar electrosurgery or preformed endoscopic ligatures to remove the tubal ectopic pregnancy and the affected tubal segment. The specimen is placed in an endoscopic specimen retrieval bag and removed through a 10 mm umbilical port.

Linear salpingostomy versus salpingectomy

The question of whether salpingostomy or salpingectomy is the superior treatment has not been studied in randomised controlled trials and is therefore still subject to debate. The drawbacks of salpingostomy – that is, the risk of persistent trophoblast and of future repeat tubal ectopic pregnancy, with the inherent medical treatment and additional costs – are justified only if this technique would result in better fertility prospects (higher spontaneous intrauterine pregnancy rate), thus reducing the cost of subsequent infertility treatment.

A review of cohort studies comparing fertility outcomes after salpingostomy and salpingectomy for tubal ectopic pregnancy showed no beneficial effect of conservative surgery on intrauterine pregnancy rates, whereas the risk of a repeat tubal ectopic pregnancy was increased, albeit not significantly.[9,10] Retrospective comparative studies reporting on life-table analysis showed a beneficial effect of salpingostomy compared with salpingectomy for tubal ectopic pregnancy in terms of future fertility prospects in women with contralateral tubal pathology and in those with previous infertility factors.[11,12]

Based on this knowledge, the RCOG guideline on the management of tubal pregnancy[13] advises performing salpingostomy in women with contralateral tubal damage, with salpingectomy being the preferred treatment in women with a healthy contralateral tube. A continuing large multicentre, international, randomised controlled trial comparing salpingectomy and salpingostomy in women diagnosed with tubal ectopic pregnancy and a normal contralateral tube at surgery (trial reference: ISRCTN37002267)should provide the definite answer to this clinical dilemma. The main outcome of interest concerns women's future fertility prospects after the index tubal ectopic pregnancy.

Complications of surgery

The complications of laparoscopic surgery are well recognised and can be minimised by the appropriate selection of women and adequate laparoscopic surgical training of the operators. Although rare, unexpected adverse events can occur during laparoscopic treatment of the tubal ectopic pregnancy, as is the case in any laparoscopic surgical procedure; however, there are certain complications that are specific to conservative surgery for tubal ectopic pregnancy.

Persistent trophoblast

Persistent tubal ectopic pregnancy can remain after a linear salpingostomy; therefore, weekly serum hCG measurements are recommended in women undergoing this procedure.[14] The incidence of persistent tubal ectopic pregnancy is higher in women who have undergone laparoscopic salpingotomy (8.5%) compared with women who have undergone a similar procedure performed at laparotomy (3.9%).[1,2]

Certain factors are associated with a higher risk of persistent trophoblast. These include higher initial serum hCG levels (>3000 iu/l), small tubal ectopic pregnancies (<20 mm in diameter) and presence of active tubal bleeding.[15]

There are expectant, medical and surgical treatment options for persistent tubal ectopic pregnancy. The choice depends on the woman's clinical symptoms and rise in hCG levels. A single dose of methotrexate (50 mg/m^2) is widely used; however, salpingectomy may become necessary in women with significant clinical symptoms or failure of serum hCG to decline.[14]

Bleeding

Bleeding is a common occurrence after linear salpingostomy. It can be controlled by ligation of blood vessels in the mesosalpinx. In women with severe bleeding, a salpingectomy can be performed as a last resort to achieve haemostasis.

Conclusion

Despite advances in ultrasound diagnosis and increasing use of conservative management of tubal ectopic pregnancy, surgery remains the most commonly used option to treat tubal ectopic pregnancy. Laparoscopic sugery has greatly improved the surgical treatment of tubal ectopic pregnancy in the last two decades, with shorter postoperative recovery times and lower costs.

However, laparotomy should still be considered in cases with signs of cardio-vascular instability. It remains unclear whether tubal conservation offers any long-term fertility benefits.

References

1 Vermesh M, Silva P D, Rosen G F, Stein A L, Fossum G T, Sauer MV. Management of unruptured ectopic gestation by linear salpingostomy: a prospective, randomized clinical trial of laparoscopy versus laparotomy. *Obstet Gynecol* 1989;73:400–4.

2 Lundorff P, Thorburn J, Hahlin M, Kallfelt B, Lindblom B. Laparoscopic surgery in ectopic pregnancy. A randomized trial versus laparotomy. *Acta Obstet Gynecol Scand* 1991;70:343–8.

3 Mol F, Mol B W, Ankum W M, van der Veen F, Hajenius P J. Current evidence on surgery, systemic methotrexate and expectant management in the treatment of tubal ectopic pregnancy: a systematic review and meta-analysis. *Hum Reprod Update* 2008;14:309–19.

4 Gray D T, Thorburn J, Lundorff P, Strandell A, Lindblom B. A cost-effectiveness study of a randomised trial of laparoscopy versus laparotomy for ectopic pregnancy. *Lancet* 1995;345:1139–43.

5 Vermesh M, Presser S C. Reproductive outcome after linear salpingostomy for ectopic gestation: a prospective 3-year follow-up. *Fertil Steril* 1992;57:682–4.

6 Lundorff P, Thorburn J, Lindblom B. Fertility outcome after conservative surgical treatment of ectopic pregnancy evaluated in a randomized trial. *Fertil Steril* 1992;57:998–1002.

7 Tulandi T, Guralnick M. Treatment of tubal ectopic pregnancy by salpingotomy with or without tubal suturing and salpingectomy. *Fertil Steril* 1991;55:53–5.

8 Fujishita A, Masuzaki H, Khan K N, Kitajima M, Hiraki K, Ishimaru T. Laparoscopic salpingotomy for tubal pregnancy: comparison of linear salpingotomy with and without suturing. *Hum Reprod* 2004;19:1195–200.

9 Clausen I. Conservative versus radical surgery for tubal pregnancy. A review. *Acta Obstet Gynecol Scand* 1996;75: 8–12.

10 Mol B W, Hajenius P J, Ankum W M, van der Veen F, Bossuyt PM. Conservative versus radical surgery for tubal pregnancy. *Acta Obstet Gynecol Scand* 1996;75:866–7.

11 Mol B W J, Matthijsse H C, Tinga D J, Huynh T, Hajenius P J, Ankum W M, et al. Fertility after conservative and radical surgery for tubal pregnancy. *Hum Reprod* 1998;13:1804–9.

12 Bouyer J, Job-Spira N, Pouly J L, Coste J, Germain E, Fernandez H. Fertility following radical, conservative-surgical or medical treatment for tubal pregnancy: a population-based study. *BJOG* 2000;107:714–21.

13 Royal College of Obstetricians and Gynaecologists. Green-top Guideline No. 21. *The management of tubal pregnancy*. London: RCOG; 2004 [www.rcog.org.uk/womens-health/clinical-guidelines/management-tubal-pregnancy-21-may-2004].

14 Hajenius P, Mol B, Ankum W M, van der Veen F, Bossuyt P M, Lammes F. Clearance curves of serum human chorionic gonadotrophin for the diagnosis of persistent trophoblast. *Hum Reprod* 1995;10:683–7.

15 Lundorff P, Hahlin M, Sjöblom P, Lindblom B. Persistent trophoblast after conservative treatment of ectopic pregnancy: prediction and detection. *Obstet Gynecol* 1991;77:129–33.

12 Diagnosis and management of non-tubal ectopic pregnancy

Davor Jurkovic and Amna Jamil

Introduction

The fallopian tube is the most common location for pregnancies that implant outside the uterine cavity. In the minds of the lay public and many health professionals, tubal implantation is often considered synonymous with ectopic pregnancy. However, there are many other locations within the pelvis and abdominal cavity where a pregnancy could implant and grow. Cases of ectopic pregnancy have been described affecting organs as distant as the liver or omentum. It has been reported that approximately 7% of all ectopic pregnancies are located outside the fallopian tubes.[1] Such pregnancies are often referred to as non-tubal ectopic pregnancies.

In recent years the incidence of ectopic pregnancy has increased owing to many factors such as improved sensitivity of urine pregnancy tests, better ultrasound diagnosis, wide use of assisted reproductive techniques and, possibly, the increased incidence of tubal damage caused by pelvic inflammatory disease. In addition, the increase in the number of surgical procedures involving the uterus, in particular the high rate of caesarean sections, has played an important role in the higher number of both tubal and non-tubal ectopic gestations.

Although non-tubal ectopic pregnancies are relatively rare, they are associated with significantly higher maternal morbidity and mortality rates compared with tubal ectopic pregnancies. This is primarily because of their tendency to remain clinically silent in early gestation and to present with acute, severe symptoms either late in the first trimester or during the second trimester of pregnancy. Clinicians are often not familiar with the diagnosis and treatment of non-tubal ectopic pregnancies, which sometimes causes delays in reaching the correct diagnosis and offering appropriate treatment.

In this chapter we describe the aetiology and risk factors for the most common types of non-tubal ectopic pregnancy. We also summarise the diagnostic criteria and describe the available management options.

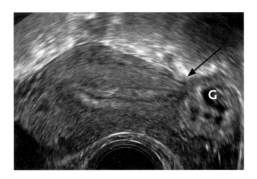

FIGURE 12.1 **Two-dimensional ultrasound scan in a woman diagnosed with an interstitial pregnancy showing a gestational sac (G) adjacent to the left lateral aspect of the uterus**

Note a continuation of the myometrial mantle surrounding the sac (arrow).

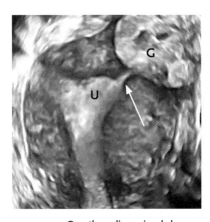

FIGURE 12.2 **On a three-dimensional planar reformatted section, the interstitial section of the tube (arrow) adjoining the uterine cavity (U) and the gestational sac (G) is clearly visible**

Interstitial pregnancy

Interstitial pregnancies occur as a result of implantation of the gestational sac in the interstitial portion of the fallopian tube. Approximately 2.5% of all ectopic pregnancies are interstitial.[1] The mortality rate associated with this condition is high, ranging from 2% to 2.5% of all cases.[2] According to the Confidential Enquiries into Maternal Deaths 2000–2002 report, there were a total of 11 deaths from ruptured ectopic pregnancy, four of which (36%) were a result of intra-abdominal haemorrhage secondary to rupture of an interstitial ectopic pregnancy.[3]

This type of ectopic pregnancy is sometimes referred to as a cornual pregnancy; however, a true cornual pregnancy is a result of implantation of a gestation in the rudimentary cornu of a unicornuate uterus, and this term should not be used to describe implantation in the intramural section of the fallopian tube. Previous tubal ectopic pregnancy, previous ipsilateral salpingectomy, sexually transmitted infections and assisted reproductive techniques are all well recognised risk factors for interstitial pregnancy.[2]

Diagnosis of interstitial pregnancy

Clinical features

Early warning signs are often absent in women with interstitial pregnancies and clinical examination is unremarkable. Women may present with sudden rupture and severe haemoperitoneum, resulting in a clinical diagnosis of ruptured ectopic pregnancy. The diagnosis of interstitial pregnancy is then established only at laparotomy or laparoscopy.

Ultrasonography

The morphological types of interstitial pregnancy vary from a gestational sac with a live embryo to a solid homogenous swelling typical of tubal miscarriage. The criteria used to establish a correct ultrasound diagnosis are listed in Box 12.1. The most useful diagnostic feature is visualisation of the interstitial section of the fallopian tube adjoining the uterine cavity and the gestational sac (Figures 12.1 and 12.2).[4] This 'interstitial line sign' is reported to have a sensitivity of 80% and specificity of 98% for the diagnosis of interstitial ectopic pregnancy. However, we believe that with a good scanning technique the diagnostic accuracy of this sign is close to 100%. Three-dimensional ultrasound facilitates visualisation of the interstitial tubes and helps to make the diagnosis in women in whom visualisation of the interstitial tubes is difficult (Figure 12.3).[5]

Other investigations

MAGNETIC RESONANCE IMAGING

The use of magnetic resonance imaging is limited to women in whom ultrasound diagnosis is uncertain. In modern clinical practice, this technique should be used only rarely for the diagnosis of interstitial ectopic pregnancy.

LAPAROSCOPY

Visualisation of a swelling at the origin of the fallopian tube lateral to the insertion of the round ligament is considered diagnostic of unruptured interstitial pregnancy at laparoscopy (Figure 12.4).[6] However, the accuracy of this finding has not been tested and a false-positive or false-negative diagnosis of interstitial pregnancy can occur in women with uterine fibroids.

Hysteroscopy should not be used for diagnostic purposes as it is not possible to visualise interstitial ectopic pregnancies using this technique. Furthermore, there is a risk of inadvertent termination of a normal intrauterine pregnancy in cases with diagnostic uncertainty.

Differential diagnosis

The differential diagnosis of a pregnancy located in the lateral aspect of the uterus includes an interstitial

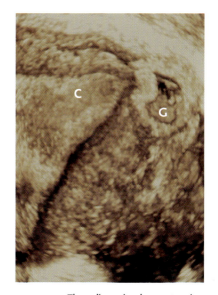

FIGURE 12.3 **Three-dimensional reconstruction of the uterine anatomy further facilitates detailed assessment of the location of the gestational sac (G) and its relation to the uterine cavity (C) and myometrium**

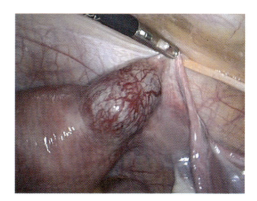

FIGURE 12.4 **A case of a right interstitial pregnancy at laparoscopy**

Note the position of the pregnancy close to the uterus without a clear surgical plane between the tubal swelling and the myometrium.

TABLE 12.1 **Criteria for differential diagnosis between intrauterine pregnancy in anomalous uteri and various forms of extrauterine pregnancy**

Type of pregnancy	Uterine shape	Number of interstitial tubes	Communication between gestational sac and uterine cavity	Continuous myometrial mantle	Mobility
Intrauterine in anomalous uterus	Abnormal	2	Wide	Yes	Absent
Tubal	Normal	2	Absent	No	Present
Interstitial	Normal	2	Narrow	Yes	Absent
Abdominal	Normal	2	Absent	No	Absent
Cornual	Abnormal	1	Absent	Yes	Present

Modified from Mavrelos et al., *Ultrasound Obstet Gynaecol*, 2007.[13]

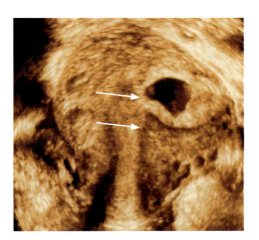

FIGURE 12.5 **A case of an intrauterine pregnancy positioned laterally in the left lateral aspect of the uterus**

A wide communication between the uterine cavity and the gestational sac (arrows) confirms the diagnosis of intrauterine pregnancy.

pregnancy, an intrauterine pregnancy located close to the tubal ostium (sometimes referred to as an angular pregnancy) and a pregnancy in an anomalous uterus. Visualisation of both interstitial tubes and the width of the communication between the gestational sac and the uterine cavity are critical features that facilitate the differential diagnosis between interstitial pregnancy and other types of ectopic pregnancy in close proximity to the uterus (Table 12.1 and Figure 12.5).

Management of interstitial pregnancy

Surgical treatment

LAPAROTOMY

Interstitial pregnancies often present late during their course owing to the surrounding thick myometrial layer and rich blood supply as a result of their close proximity to the uterus.[2] Additional delays can be caused by difficulties in reaching the correct diagnosis. As a result, cornual resection at laparotomy or hysterectomy because of uncontrolled haemorrhage was often the treatment received by women presenting with significant intra-abdominal bleeding.

LAPAROSCOPY

Early non-invasive ultrasound diagnosis prior to the rupture facilitates the use of laparoscopic surgery for the treatment of interstitial ectopic pregnancy.

Various procedures have been described, including laparoscopic cornual resection, cornuostomy and salpingotomy.[7] Intramyometrial vasopressin injection and a suture-loop tourniquet through a broad ligament have been used to reduce intraoperative blood loss. Intraoperative haemorrhage is usually caused by attempts at partial resection of the fundal myometrium, which is performed to achieve complete removal of the ectopic trophoblast. Cornual resection can also result in focal myometrial deficiency, which increases the risk of uterine rupture in future pregnancies.

At University College Hospital, London (UCHL), an alternative approach has been developed to avoid performing cornual resection in women with interstitial pregnancy. To achieve this we inject the interstitial ectopic pregnancy with methotrexate before the laparoscopy. The procedure is performed under ultrasound guidance and the medication is administered directly into the gestational sac. During the operation a suture loop is inserted around the bulging interstitial ectopic pregnancy. The suture is then tied and the bulging myometrium is incised to remove as much of the trophoblast as possible. Trophoblastic tissue below the suture line can be left to resolve spontaneously as it has already been treated with methotrexate (Figures 12.6 and 12.7).

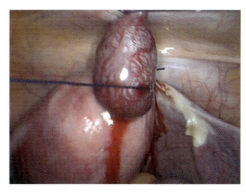

FIGURE 12.6 **Laparoscopic treatment of interstitial pregnancy using an endoloop, which is placed as close to the uterus as possible**

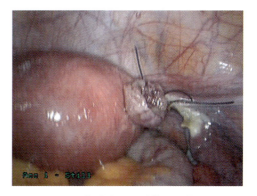

FIGURE 12.7 **Small tubal stump following the excision of pregnancy**

Any remaining trophoblast tissue below the suture line can be treated with methotrexate.

Conservative management

MEDICAL TREATMENT

Methotrexate, a folic acid antagonist, is a widely used treatment option in women who are haemodynamically stable with unruptured interstitial ectopic pregnancies. In general, smaller pregnancies with lower serum human chorionic gonadotrophin (hCG) levels at the initial presentation have a better chance of being treated successfully with methotrexate.[8]

Methotrexate can be administered systemically in single or multiple doses. Alternatively, local administration in the ectopic sac under ultrasound guidance is increasingly being used owing to its higher efficacy (91% compared with 79% with systemic methotrexate) and fewer adverse effects.[7] The technique of local administration has previously been described.[8] The vagina

FIGURE 12.8 The conservative management of interstitial ectopic pregnancies

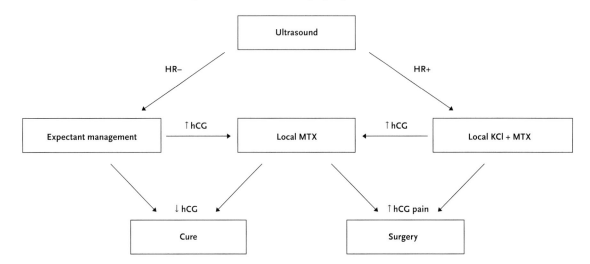

hCG = human chorionic gonadotrophin | HR = heart rate | KCl = potassium chloride | MTX = methotrexate.

is cleansed using an antiseptic solution such as 0.015% chlorhexidine, and antibiotic cover is given (cefuroxime 750 mg intravenously or metronidazole 500 mg intravenously). A 20-gauge spinal needle is placed into a needle guide and advanced through the anterior vaginal fornix and anterior uterine wall into the gestational sac. Exocoelomic fluid is aspirated first and 25 mg of methotrexate is injected into the coelomic cavity. In viable pregnancies an embryocide should be performed first by injecting 0.2–0.4 mEq of potassium chloride intracardially.

EXPECTANT MANAGEMENT

Expectant management is suitable for women who are stable with non-viable interstitial pregnancies and declining hCG levels. Serial monitoring of hCG levels is continued until the level becomes undetectable. Approximately 20% of all interstitial ectopic pregnancies are considered suitable for expectant management, with 70% of those pregnancies resolving spontaneously during follow-up.[8] A flow chart illustrating the management of interstitial pregnancies at UCHL is provided in Figure 12.8.

UTERINE ARTERY EMBOLISATION

Selective uterine artery embolisation is sometimes used to treat or prevent heavy bleeding during surgical treatment of interstitial pregnancy. Its use after failure of conservative treatment with systemic methotrexate has also been described.[9]

Fertility after interstitial pregnancy

There is a paucity of data regarding future reproductive outcomes following treatment of interstitial pregnancy. A study by Sawyer et al.[10] reported spontaneous conception in the majority of women and a recurrence of ectopic pregnancy in 23% of cases. Two-thirds of recurrent ectopic pregnancies were interstitial and the remaining third were tubal.

Cervical and caesarean-scar pregnancies

Cervical and caesarean-scar pregnancies are similar in their aetiology, pathophysiology and clinical presentation. They are both caused by previous surgical trauma to the uterus. Cervical pregnancies are usually implanted into a myometrial defect caused by a false passage, which sometimes occurs during difficult cervical dilatation. Caesarean-scar pregnancies are the result of the pregnancy implanting into a deficient lower-uterine-segment caesarean section scar. As a result, both cervical and caesarean pregnancies have a tendency to penetrate deep into the myometrium. This is the main reason, rather than their location outside the uterine cavity, for their propensity to cause severe bleeding during spontaneous or surgical evacuation.[11] Cervical pregnancies are relatively rare, accounting for fewer than 1% of all ectopic gestations.[12] Caesarean-scar pregnancies are more common, occurring in one in 1800 pregnancies.

Diagnosis of cervical and caesarean-scar pregnancies

Clinical features
Painless vaginal bleeding is the most common presenting symptom of cervical and caesarean-scar pregnancies. In advanced cases, the bleeding can be associated with abdominal pain and urinary symptoms.[13] Findings on clinical examination are variable and may include visualisation of an enlarged cervix or bulging lower uterine segment. The cervix is often open.[12]

Ultrasonography
Historically, the diagnosis of cervical pregnancy was made on histological examination of the uterus following a hysterectomy to control severe haemorrhage. Since 1978, when the first sonographic report of cervical pregnancy

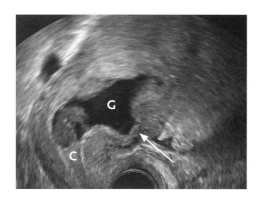

FIGURE 12.9 **A case of caesarean-scar pregnancy at 7 weeks of gestation**

The sac (G) is implanted into a large anterior myometrial defect (arrow). Note that the cervix is already open (C), which indicates that the pregnancy is unlikely to progress much further.

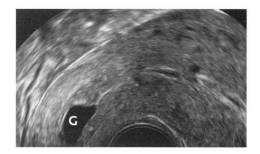

FIGURE 12.10 **A case of a small cervical pregnancy (G), implanted low in the posterior aspect of the cervix**

was published, ultrasound has become the mainstay of diagnosis of this rare form of pregnancy.[14] The morphological types of cervical pregnancy can vary from a haemorrhagic mass to a gestational sac with an embryo, with or without cardiac activity.[12]

Until recently, early caesarean scar pregnancies could not be differentiated from cervical pregnancies. It is therefore not surprising that in the past a history of previous caesarean section was considered to be one of the main risk factors for cervical implantation. Caesarean-scar pregnancies are typically located close to the internal os, in contrast to cervical pregnancies, which tend to be located lower in the cervix (Figures 12.9 and 12.10). As a result, caesarean-scar pregnancies are more likely to contain a live embryo and to progress into the second trimester and occasionally to full term, which makes them more difficult to manage than cervical pregnancies.

Differential diagnosis

Differential diagnosis between cervical and caesarean-scar pregnancies is possible only on transvaginal ultrasound scan. However, this is of little importance as the management of both types of pregnancy is similar. Caesarean-scar pregnancies that are located high at the internal os may progress to full term and some women may therefore opt for expectant management in the hope that the fetus will reach viability. The risk of late miscarriage and early preterm delivery is very high in these women and expectant management should be contemplated only after detailed counselling about the potential risks to the mother and baby. The ultrasound criteria used at UCHL for the diagnosis of cervical and scar pregnancies are described in Box 12.2.[15,16] These criteria enable differential diagnosis between a true extrauterine implantation and the cervical phase of a spontaneous miscarriage of an intrauterine pregnancy. In cases of miscarriage, the gestational sac is mobile on palpation with no evidence of trophoblastic flow (Figures 12.11 and 12.12).

Additional diagnostic pitfalls may occur when the pregnancy is implanted in the lower part of the uterine corpus. In these cases it may be difficult to achieve sonographic differentiation of the endocervical canal from the isthmic portion of the uterine cavity. This is even harder after the first trimester of pregnancy. In a coronal view of the uterus, the level of insertion of the uterine artery may be a helpful clue to determine the level of the internal os.[17] However, the critical feature is the penetration of the pregnancy in the myometrium, which is easier to assess early in the first trimester.

Management of cervical and caesarean-scar pregnancies

Traditionally, cervical pregnancies were treated with hysterectomy, owing to late presentation which was often caused by severe vaginal bleeding. Hysterectomy remains the treatment of choice in women with advanced cervical pregnancies complicated with life-threatening haemorrhage. The introduction of high-frequency vaginal transducers has led to diagnosis earlier in the pregnancy, when the risk of bleeding is lower and conservative medical and surgical options can be used successfully. Since the introduction of ultrasound scanning, the rate of emergency hysterectomy for cervical pregnancy has decreased to 15%, and in modern practice it is very rare that hysterectomy is required to control the bleeding.

Caesarean-scar pregnancies are more likely to remain clinically silent until later in pregnancy, when they tend to evolve into placenta praevia accreta/percreta.[18] In these pregnancies, caesarean hysterectomy is often required following delivery of the fetus.

Surgical management

Dilatation and curettage is the main surgical treatment modality for cervical and caesarean-scar pregnancies. Owing to myometrial involvement, the removal of the pregnancy may be associated with uncontrolled bleeding.[15] As a result, a number of adjunctive methods to control intraoperative bleeding have been described. These include insertion of a Foley catheter in the cervix for 24–48 hours, intracervical vasopressin injection, cervical Shirodkar cerclage, transvaginal ligation

BOX 12.2 **Sonographic criteria for diagnosis of cervical and caesarean-scar pregnancy**

- Presence of gestational sac or placental tissue below or at the level of the internal os

- Clear evidence of pregnancy invading into the myometrium

- Evidence of sustained peritrophoblastic circulation on colour Doppler examination, characterised by high blood-flow velocity (over 20 cm/sec) and low impedance (PI <1) circulation

- Negative sliding organ sign (inability to displace the gestational sac from its position using gentle pressure with a transvaginal probe)

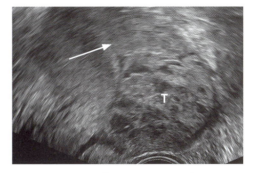

FIGURE 12.11 **A case of caesarean-scar ectopic pregnancy**

Trophoblast (T) is seen within the anterior wall of the uterus, below the uterine cavity (arrow).

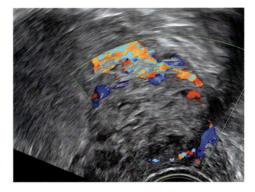

FIGURE 12.12 **Demonstration of high vascular supply on Doppler examination facilitates the differential diagnosis between cervical phase of miscarriage**

of the cervical branches of the uterine arteries and angiographic uterine artery embolisation. UCHL favours insertion of a cervical suture, which is an excellent method of controlling bleeding after evacuation of cervical and caesarean-scar pregnancies. In advanced cases a local injection of metrotrexate 1 week before evacuation can be used to facilitate separation of the trophoblast from the myometrium and reduce the risk of incomplete evacuation of the pregnancy.[19]

Medical management

Systemic methotrexate in single- or multiple-dose regimens is the most widely used chemotherapeutic agent for the treatment of tubal ectopic pregnancies. Its successful use has also been reported in cervical and caesarean-scar pregnancies.[11,15] However, many women experience serious adverse effects after administration of methotrexate.

Transvaginal local injection of methotrexate under ultrasound guidance is easy to administer owing to the proximity of the pregnancy to the vagina and the thick layer of myometrium surrounding cervical and caesarean-scar pregnancies. The main advantages of local injection are the use of a much lower dose of the drug with a reduction in adverse effects and greater efficacy.

Although medical treatment is effective in arresting trophoblastic proliferation, it often takes many months for the pregnancy tissue to become absorbed. During this time women tend to bleed intermittently and often heavily, which prevents them from resuming their normal social and professional activities. These problems limit the use of conservative medical treatment in the management of cervical and caesarean-scar pregnancies.

The optimal approach to the treatment of cervical and caesarean-scar pregnancies is determined by several factors, the most important of which are clinical symptoms, gestational age and presence of cardiac activity. A flow chart illustrating the management of cervical and caesarean scar pregnancy at UCHL is provided in Figure 12.13.

Fertility after cervical and caesarean-scar pregnancies

The recurrence rate of cervical pregnancy is only 3%; however, it has been reported to be associated with an increased risk of tubal pregnancy and preterm delivery.[11] The recurrence rate of caesarean-scar pregnancy is 1–2% and the rate of spontaneous conception after successful treatment is as high as 86%.[20] It is recommended to delay subsequent pregnancies for up to 3 months to promote scar healing.[21]

FIGURE 12.13 **The management of caesarean-scar and cervical ectopic pregnancies at less than 14 weeks of gestation**

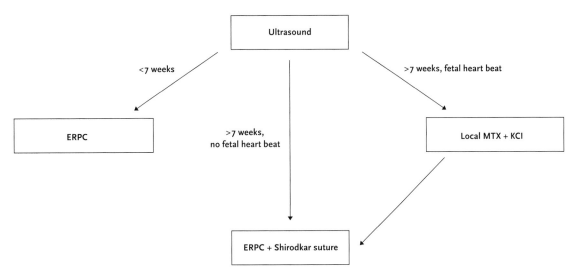

ERPC = evacuation of retained products of conception | KCl = potassium chloride | MTX = methotrexate.

Ovarian pregnancy

Ovarian pregnancy is the result of the conceptus implanting inside or on the surface of the ovary. It accounts for approximately 3% of all ectopic pregnancies.[1,22] Risk factors are similar to those for tubal ectopic pregnancies and include pelvic inflammatory disease, previous ectopic pregnancy, endometriosis, intrauterine contraceptive device use and assisted conception.[23]

Diagnosis of ovarian pregnancy

The clinical presentation of ovarian pregnancy usually resembles that of tubal pregnancy. Ultrasound is the first-line investigation for non-invasive diagnosis. It involves visualisation of the following features, which enable a correct preoperative diagnosis to be reached:

- presence of a cystic structure with an echogenic ring surrounded by healthy ovarian tissue and separate from the corpus luteum

- inability to separate the gestational sac from the ovary on gentle palpation (negative sliding organ sign).

Visualisation of the corpus luteum separate from the ovarian pregnancy is essential. This avoids mistaking a cystic corpus for an ovarian pregnancy (Figure

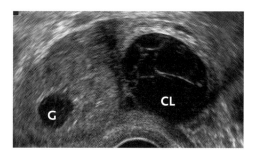

FIGURE 12.14 **A case of an ovarian pregnancy (G)** located adjacent to a corpus luteum (CL)

12.14). A negative sliding organ sign is not entirely specific and can occasionally be observed in tubal ectopic pregnancies that are fixed to the ipsilateral ovary by pelvic adhesions. A definite ultrasound diagnosis can be difficult to achieve in some women, especially in those presenting with rupture.

At surgery, the ovarian pregnancy is seen as a swelling in the ovary separate from the corpus luteum with normal fallopian tubes. The diagnosis can be confirmed histologically by the presence of ovarian tissue adjacent to the gestational sac.

Management of ovarian pregnancy

Laparoscopic ovarian resection, removal of the products of conception with biopsy forceps and hydrodissection are the commonly used conservative surgical methods in the management of ovarian pregnancy. All of these techniques allow preservation of the ovarian tissue and of fertility.[24] Ovarian wedge resection at laparotomy or oophorectomy is sometimes required in women with large ovarian pregnancies with significant intraperitoneal bleeding.

Cornual pregnancy

Cornual pregnancy is one of the rarest forms of ectopic pregnancy, with an incidence of 1/76 000 pregnancies.[25] It occurs as a result of implantation of the conceptus in a rudimentary horn of a unicornuate uterus, which is a rare congenital anomaly that occurs in approximately 0.3% of women. Nearly 75% of unicornuate uteri have an accessory horn, which may or may not communicate with the uterine cavity.[26] The majority of rudimentary horns contain functional endometrium and are non-communicating. The implantation of the pregnancy in such cases is thought to occur as a result of transperitoneal migration of sperm and fertilisation in the ipsilateral fallopian tube.

Diagnosis of cornual pregnancy

Clinical features

In contrast to tubal ectopic pregnancies, cornual pregnancies mostly follow an early asymptomatic course and can remain unrecognised until the second trimester of pregnancy. There is a significant health risk to women with

BOX 12.3 **Sonographic criteria for diagnosis of cornual pregnancies**

○ Empty uterine cavity with a single interstitial fallopian tube

○ Gestational sac separate from the uterus and completely surrounded by myometrium

○ Positive sliding organ sign

○ Vascular pedicle adjoining the gestational sac with the unicornuate uterus

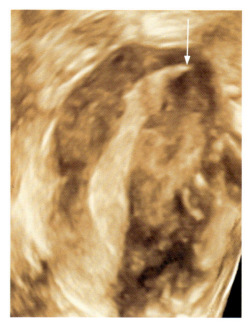

FIGURE 12.15 **An example of unicornuate uterus on three-dimensional ultrasound scan**

Note the narrow uterine cavity, which deviates to the left with a single interstitial tube at the fundus (arrow).

cornual pregnancies, as 50% of such pregnancies are liable to uterine rupture and severe intraperitoneal bleeding. The majority of such events occur during the second trimester. More recently, with improved diagnosis and early intervention, the maternal mortality rate associated with cornual pregnancies has significantly decreased. However, the morbidity rate remains considerably higher, as 50% of cornual pregnancies are diagnosed only after uterine rupture.[25]

Ultrasonography

There are clear ultrasound criteria that enable an accurate diagnosis of cornual pregnancies and facilitate their differentiation from other forms of ectopic pregnancy (Box 12.3). It is imperative to differentiate cornual pregnancies from interstitial ectopic pregnancies. The clinical course and management strategies for the two types differ markedly, so an accurate diagnosis is essential for planning appropriate treatment. The presence of an empty uterine cavity with a single interstitial tube adjacent to the ectopic gestational sac is a pathognomic feature of a cornual pregnancy and is consistently found even at advanced gestation (Figures 12.15 and 12.16). Mobility of the gestational sac and the presence of a vascular pedicle are other distinctive features.[27]

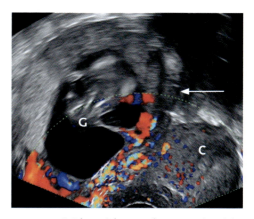

FIGURE 12.16 **A large right cornual pregnancy in a right non-communicating uterine cornu (G)**

Note the presence of thick myometrium surrounding the gestational sac (arrow) and extensive blood supply at the medial aspect of the sac. C = left cornu.

Other investigations

In recent years three-dimensional ultrasonography has become the method of choice for the diagnosis of congenital uterine anomalies. This technique is particularly helpful for the differential diagnosis between a unicornuate uterus and other types of congenital uterine anomalies. The use of magnetic resonance imaging should be reserved for women with an uncertain diagnosis where three-dimensional scanning is not available.

To minimise the risk of intraoperative urological complications, it is vital to perform a thorough examination of the genitourinary system to exclude concomitant urological anomalies before planning surgical treatment.

Differential diagnosis of cornual pregnancy

Tubal ectopic pregnancies usually follow an acute course and are rarely found beyond the first trimester. Interstitial and abdominal ectopic pregnancies are therefore included among the important differential diagnoses of cornual pregnancies later in the course of pregnancy. The interstitial line sign, as previously described, is a useful marker to differentiate interstitial pregnancies from cornual pregnancies. Additionally, unlike cornual pregnancies, interstitial ectopic pregnancies are not mobile and they are surrounded by a myometrial mantle that is continuous with the uterine musculature. Abdominal pregnancies also differ as they lack the myometrial mantle and tend to be fixed deeply in the pelvis.

Management of cornual pregnancy

The choice of management option for cornual pregnancies should be made on an individual basis. Owing to the high rate of rupture of these pregnancies and the resulting maternal morbidity associated with intraperitoneal bleeding, surgical removal of the pregnancy along with excision of the rudimentary horn is considered the treatment of choice as soon as the diagnosis is established. Expectant management and a careful approach to continuation of the pregnancy have been reported in selected cases when the diagnosis has been made in asymptomatic women late in the second or early in the third trimester of pregnancy. However, the risk of rupture remains high and the pregnancy should be concluded when the fetus has a good chance of survival.

Surgical management

Surgical treatment of cornual pregnancy involves excision of the rudimentary horn by division of the vascular pedicle between the pregnancy and the uterus. Some authors have advocated the use of methotrexate or feticide with potassium chloride prior to surgical treatment in an attempt to reduce intraoperative blood loss.[28,29]

The surgical approach is largely determined by the clinical urgency and the level of expertise of the laparoscopic surgeon. There are several case reports of successful laparoscopic surgical treatment of cornual pregnancies in recent years. The division of the vascular pedicle is achieved by using electrosurgery or stapling devices, and the rudimentary cornu and the pregnancy are removed via posterior colpotomy or suprapubic incision using a morcellator.[29]

Despite the obvious advantages of laparoscopy in terms of faster recovery and shorter hospital stay, laparotomy remains the preferred approach in women with uterine rupture and women who are diagnosed late in the second trimester.

Expectant management

With the improvements in fetal survival achieved over the last few decades, cornual pregnancies diagnosed late in the second trimester can occasionally be managed conservatively and delivered when fetal viability is achieved. In the largest series of rudimentary horn pregnancies, approximately 30% of cases continued to develop until term, suggesting that progression of pregnancies can occur in selected cases.[25] However, owing to the continuing risk of sudden rupture, women should be managed on an inpatient basis until delivery. There is little advantage of allowing these pregnancies to progress beyond 32 weeks of gestation. Delivery should be by elective surgery, which should always include excision of the rudimentary cornu.

Fertility after cornual pregnancy

Surgical treatment of cornual pregnancy usually involves removal of the rudimentary cornu, which prevents further recurrence. However, the risk of recurrence is likely to be high after conservative management. In a series of six women studied by Mavrelos et al.,[27] one woman who was managed conservatively had a recurrent cornual pregnancy 1 year later.

Abdominal pregnancy

Abdominal pregnancy occurs as a result of implantation of the gestational sac in the peritoneal cavity, outside the uterus, ovaries and fallopian tubes. It accounts for 1% of all ectopic pregnancies and is associated with significantly higher mortality figures compared with tubal ectopic pregnancies.[1,30]

Two subtypes of abdominal pregnancy have been described. Primary abdominal pregnancy occurs when the primary implantation site is the peritoneal cavity. Secondary abdominal pregnancy, which is much more common, is the result of tubal abortion and reimplantation into the abdominal cavity. In these cases the trophoblast penetrates through the wall of the tube and invades the surrounding organs. The most common location of abdominal pregnancy is the broad ligament. Rich vascularity within the broad ligament can provide sufficient support to the pregnancy to enable it to develop to full term.

Diagnosis of abdominal pregnancy

The appearance of an early abdominal pregnancy on ultrasonography is characterised by an empty uterine cavity and the presence of a gestational sac or trophoblastic mass separate from the uterus, adnexa and ovaries. Differential diagnosis between abdominal, tubal and ovarian pregnancy can be difficult in early pregnancy. In late gestation, abnormal fetal lie, oligohydramnios and signs of placental insufficiency are often present in women with abdominal pregnancies.[31]

Management of abdominal pregnancy

The management of early abdominal pregnancy is relatively simple and can be achieved using the laparoscopic approach.[32] Traditional management of advanced abdominal pregnancy involves laparotomy and delivery of the fetus. The placenta should be left in place if at all possible, as attempts to remove it are likely to result in severe uncontrollable haemorrhage. Both approaches have been used in conjunction with administration of methotrexate and selective arterial embolisation to minimise the risk of severe haemorrhage. However, the value of methotrexate in women with advanced abdominal pregnancy is not clear.

Conclusion

Non-tubal ectopic pregnancies represent an important challenge to clinicians who provide care to women with suspected early pregnancy complications. Non-tubal ectopic pregnancies are relatively rare and it is difficult for individual practitioners to develop wide experience in their diagnosis and management. Diagnostic errors and delays increase the risk of adverse outcomes as advanced cases are more difficult to manage than those diagnosed early in the first trimester of pregnancy. Therefore, all consultants in early pregnancy care should be familiar with the principles of diagnosis and management. When the diagnosis is uncertain, or when the diagnosis is made late in the first trimester or during the second trimester, referral to a tertiary centre should be considered.

References

1 Bouyer J, Coste J, Fernandez H, Pouly J L, Job-Spira N. Sites of ectopic pregnancy: a 10 year population-based study of 1800 cases. *Hum Reprod* 2002;17:3224–30.

2 Tulandi T, Al-Jaroudi D. Interstitial pregnancy: results generated from the Society of Reproductive Surgeons Registry. *Obstet Gynecol* 2004;103:47–50.

3 Lewis P G, editor. *Why Mothers Die 2000–2002 – The Sixth Report of Confidential Enquiries into Maternal Deaths in the United Kingdon*. London: RCOG Press; 2004.

4 Ackerman T E, Levi C S, Dashefsky S M, Holt S C, Lindsay D J. Interstitial line: sonographic finding in interstitial (cornual) ectopic pregnancy. *Radiology* 1993;189:83–7.

5 Lawrence A, Jurkovic D. Three-dimensional ultrasound diagnosis of interstitial pregnancy. *Ultrasound Obstet Gynecol* 1999;14:292–3.

6 Jansen R P, Elliott P M. Angular intrauterine pregnancy. *Obstet Gynecol* 1981;58:167–75.

7 Lau S, Tulandi T. Conservative medical and surgical management of interstitial ectopic pregnancy. *Fertil Steril* 1999;72:207–15.

8 Cassik P, Ofili-Yebovi D, Yazbek J, Lee C, Elson J, Jurkovic D. Factors influencing the success of conservative treatment of interstitial pregnancy. *Ultrasound Obstet Gynecol* 2005;26:279–82.

9 Ophir E, Singer-Jordan J, Oettinger M, Odeh M, Tendler R, Feldman Y, et al. Uterine artery embolization for management of interstitial twin ectopic pregnancy: case report. *Hum Reprod* 2004;19:1774–7.

10 Helmy S, Sawyer E, Ofili-Yebovi D, Yazbek J, Ben Nagi J, Jurkovic D. Fertility outcomes following expectant management of tubal ectopic pregnancy. *Ultrasound Obstet Gynecol* 2007;30:988–93.

11 Benson C B, Doubilet P M. Strategies for conservative treatment of cervical ectopic pregnancy. *Ultrasound Obstet Gynecol* 1996;8:371–2.

12 Ushakov F B, Elchalal U, Aceman P J, Schenker J G. Cervical pregnancy: past and future. *Obstet Gynecol Surv* 1997;52:45–59.

13 Copas P, Semmer J. Cervical ectopic pregnancy: sonographic demonstration at twenty-eight weeks gestation. *J Clin Ultrasound* 1983;11:328–30.

14 Raskin M M. Diagnosis of cervical pregnancy by ultrasound: a case report. *Am J Obstet Gynecol* 1978;130:234–5.

15 Jurkovic D, Hacket E, Campbell S. Diagnosis and treatment of early cervical pregnancy: a review and a report of two cases treated conservatively. *Ultrasound Obstet Gynecol* 1996;8:373–80.

16 Vial Y, Petignat P, Hohlfeld P. Pregnancy in a cesarean scar. *Ultrasound Obstet Gynecol* 2000;16:592–3.

17 Timor-Tritsch I E, Monteagudo A, Mandeville E O, Peisner D B, Anaya G P, Pirrone E C. Successful management of viable cervical pregnancy by local injection of methotrexate guided by transvaginal ultrasonography. *Am J Obstet Gynecol* 1994;170:737–9.

18 Ben Nagi J, Ofili-Yebovi D, Marsh M, Jurkovic D. First-trimester cesarean scar pregnancy evolving into placenta previa/accreta at term. *J Ultrasound Med* 2005;24:1569–73.

19 Jurkovic D, Ben-Nagi J, Ofilli-Yebovi D, Sawyer E, Helmy S, Yazbek J. Efficacy of Shirodkar cervical suture in securing haemostasis following surgical evacuation of Cesarean scar ectopic pregnancy. *Ultrasound Obstet Gynecol* 2007;30:95–100.

20 Ben Nagi J, Helmy S, Ofili-Yebovi D, Yazbek J, Sawyer E, Jurkovic D. Reproductive outcomes of women with a previous history of Caesarean scar ectopic pregnancies. *Hum Reprod* 2007;22:2012–15.

21 Seow K M, Huang L W, Lin Y H, Lin M Y, Tsai Y L, Hwang J L. Cesarean scar pregnancy: issues in management. *Ultrasound Obstet Gynecol* 2004;23:247–53.

22 Gaudoin M R, Coulter KL, Robins A M, Verghese A, Hanretty K P. Is the incidence of ovarian ectopic pregnancy increasing? *Eur J Obstet Gynecol Reprod Biol* 1996;70:141–3.

23 Raziel A, Schachter M, Mordechai E, Friedler S, Panski M, Ron-El R. Ovarian pregnancy—a 12-year experience of 19 cases in one institution. *Eur J Obstet Gynecol Reprod Biol* 2004;114:92–6.

24 Seinera P, Di Gregorio A, Arisio R, Decko A, Crana F. Ovarian pregnancy and operative laparoscopy: a report of eight cases. *Hum Reprod* 1997;12:608–10.

25 Nahum G G. Rudimentary uterine horn pregnancy. The 20th-century worldwide experience of 588 cases. *J Reprod Med* 2002;47:151–63.

26 Jayasinghe Y, Rane A, Stalewski H, Grover S. The presentation and early diagnosis of the rudimentary uterine horn. *Obstet Gynecol* 2005;105:1456–67.

27 Mavrelos D, Sawyer E, Helmy S, Holland T K, Ben-Nagi J, Jurkovic D. Ultrasound diagnosis of ectopic pregnancy in the non-communicating horn of a unicornuate uterus (cornual pregnancy). *Ultrasound Obstet Gynecol* 2007;30:765–70.

28 Edelman A B, Jensen J T, Lee D M, Nichols M D. Successful medical abortion of a pregnancy within a noncommunicating rudimentary uterine horn. *Am J Obstet Gynecol* 2003;189: 886–7.

29 Cutner A, Saridogan E, Hart R, Pandya P, Creighton S. Laparoscopic management of pregnancies occurring in non-communicating accessory uterine horns. *Eur J Obstet Gynecol Reprod Biol* 2004;113:106–9.

30 Atrash H K, Friede A, Hogue C J. Abdominal pregnancy in the United States: frequency and maternal mortality. *Obstet Gynecol* 1987;69:333–7.

31 Kwok A, Chia K K, Ford R, Lam A. Laparoscopic management of a case of abdominal ectopic pregnancy. *Aust N Z J Obstet Gynaecol* 2002:42:300–2.

32 Rahaman J, Berkowitz R, Mitty H, Gaddipati S, Brown B, Nezhat F. Minimally invasive management of an advanced abdominal pregnancy. *Obstet Gynecol* 2004;103:1064–8.

13 Diagnosis and management of acute pelvic pain

Jackie Ross

Introduction

Acute pelvic pain is usually defined as pain of less than 2 weeks' duration. While this chapter focuses on the common gynaecological conditions that cause acute pain, it should be borne in mind that a woman may suffer an acute exacerbation of a chronic condition that may or may not have been previously diagnosed. Therefore, in some women the cause of the acute pain will be a condition typically associated with chronic pelvic pain. This chapter primarily describes the clinical approach to the management of acute pelvic pain rather than providing detailed descriptions of separate pathological entities causing pain. The emphasis is on clinical presentation and differential diagnosis of pelvic pain, with plenty of practical advice.

History and clinical examination

Taking a detailed history is one of the most important elements of the clinical assessment of a woman presenting with acute pelvic pain. Even if you are not the first person to see the woman and her history has already been taken by a colleague, it is always worth hearing the woman describe the onset and character of the pain again in her own words. The uterus, cervix and adnexa share the same visceral innervation as the lower ileum, sigmoid colon and rectum. Afferent pain signals travel via the sympathetic nerves to spinal cord segments T10 to L1. Because of this shared pathway, distinguishing between pain of gynaecological origin and pain of gastrointestinal origin is often difficult. Acute pain owing to ischaemia or injury to a viscus is accompanied by autonomic reflex responses such as nausea, vomiting, restlessness and sweating. Once the overlying peritoneum becomes inflamed or irritated, the pain stimuli are transmitted by the same somatic nerves used by the overlying skin. As a result, the pain becomes better localised and sharper in character. Figures 13.1–13.4 show the patterns of pain typically associated with the common causes of acute pelvic pain.

FIGURE 13.1 **Typical pattern of pain associated with inflammation such as pelvic inflammatory disease**

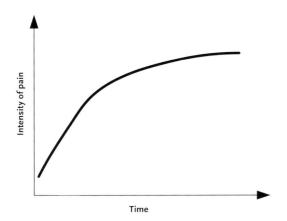

FIGURE 13.2 **Typical pattern of pain associated with a haemorrhagic or ruptured functional ovarian cyst**

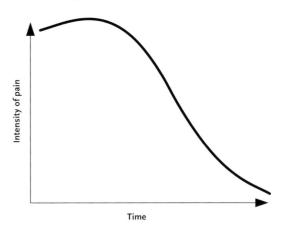

FIGURE 13.3 **Typical pattern of pain associated with ovarian torsion or renal colic**

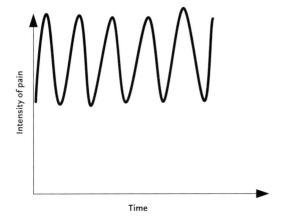

FIGURE 13.4 **Typical pattern of pain associated with uterine or gastrointestinal pathology**

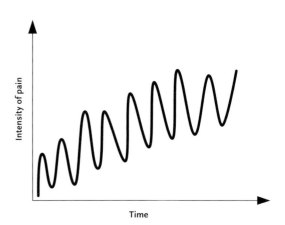

The potential causes of acute pelvic pain are listed in Table 13.1. In sexually active women it is often difficult to differentiate between acute pelvic inflammatory disease (PID) and appendicitis. Clinical features that favour the diagnosis of PID are non-migratory pain, bilateral pelvic tenderness and absence of nausea or vomiting. In a retrospective study, diarrhoea, fever and rebound tenderness were not found to be helpful in the differential diagnosis.[1] The Centers for Disease Control and Prevention criteria for the diagnosis of acute PID are shown in Table 13.2.[2] The minimal criteria alone are highly sensitive but relatively non-specific for the diagnosis of PID.[3] This can result

TABLE 13.1 **Causes of acute pelvic pain**

Gynaecological causes	Pregnancy-related causes	Nongynaecological causes
Salpingitis/pelvic inflammatory disease	Ectopic pregnancy	Appendicitis
Tubo-ovarian abscess	Uterine contractions	Mesenteric adenitis
Ovulation pain	Placental abruption	Irritable bowel syndrome
Haemorrhage into or from the corpus luteum	Fibroid degeneration	Constipation
Ruptured ovarian cyst	Uterine rupture	Inflammatory bowel disease
Ovarian torsion	Incarcerated retroverted uterus	Meckel's diverticulum
Ovarian hyperstimulation syndrome		Diverticulitis
Dysmenorrhoea		Mesenteric infarction
Haematometra		Intussusception
Torsion/rupture of fibroid		Hernia
		Urinary infection
		Renal colic
		Acute urinary retention
		Aortic aneurysm
		Porphyria

in overtreatment with antibiotics. However, it has been suggested that the benefits gained by preventing the long-term complications of untreated PID outweigh the risks of adverse effects from antibiotic therapy, particularly in young nulliparous women.[2,3] Both intraperitoneal haemorrhage and ovarian torsion[4] may be associated with low-grade pyrexia, so one should be wary of

TABLE 13.2 **Centers for Disease Control and Prevention criteria for the diagnosis of acute PID[2]**

Minimal criteria	Additional criteria
Uterine tenderness	Temperature higher than 101°F (38.3°C)
Adnexal tenderness	Abnormal cervical or vaginal mucopurulent discharge
Cervical excitation	Presence of white blood cells on saline microscopy of vaginal secretions
	Elevated erythrocyte sedimentation rate
	Elevated C-reactive protein level
	Laboratory documentation of cervical infection with *Neisseria gonorrhoea* or *Chlamydia trachomatis*

considering fever as a conclusive sign of pelvic infection without considering other causes.

The typical history of sudden-onset, stabbing, sharp pain should raise the suspicion of haemorrhage from a functional cyst. The pain will become dull and less severe over the following 2–3 days. It is also worth remembering that haemorrhagic cysts tend to occur in women with natural menstrual cycles, that is women not using forms of contraception that cause ovarian suppression such as the combined oral contraceptive pill[5] and injectables. The risk factors for excessive haemorrhage into functional cysts are the presence of endometriosis or pelvic adhesions, bleeding diatheses and anticoagulation therapy.[6] In general terms, uncomplicated functional ovarian cysts cause pain only if they grow very quickly and cause rapid distension of the ovarian capsule. True ovarian cysts tend to grow slowly and therefore can become very large without causing pelvic pain.

Ovarian torsion is a far less common cause of acute pelvic pain and is said to account for only 2% of emergency admissions.[7] Nausea and vomiting are associated with the pain of torsion in 85% of cases.[8] The heavier and more mobile the ovary, the more likely it is to twist, so women with dermoid cysts or polycystic ovaries are particularly prone to ovarian torsion. Acute pain occurring in young girls or postmenopausal women is more likely to be a result of torsion than is acute pain occurring in women in the reproductive age group. This is because functional haemorrhagic cysts, which are a common cause of pain in the fertile years, do not usually occur in the absence of ovarian activity.

Women with ovarian hyperstimulation syndrome will usually report a history of recent ovarian stimulation, most commonly with injected gonadotrophins but occasionally with clomifene. Rare cases have been reported in association with spontaneous pregnancies.[9]

Acute pelvic pain of uterine origin is unusual. Fibroids rarely undergo painful degeneration outside pregnancy, although they may very occasionally undergo torsion or rupture. Cyclical pain in association with secondary amenorrhoea may be the result of haematometra; if this is the case, there is usually a history of preceding uterine instrumentation such as a surgical termination of pregnancy or colposcopic surgery. Haematometra may also be the result of a non-communicating rudimentary horn but, in these cases, women typically present with a history of primary dysmenorrhoea and may go on to develop secondary severe endometriosis owing to retrograde menstruation.[10]

Laboratory tests

Simple urinalysis is usually the first test performed in women with acute pelvic pain. This test is often performed by the triage nurse in the emergency department. Microscopic haematuria has been reported as a useful test in adult women with pain radiating to the flank or loin, as it is present in 80–100% of those with confirmed renal colic caused by stones. However, the specificity may be as low as 30%.[11] Most studies looking at the usefulness of urinalysis have not specifically tested women presenting with acute abdominal or pelvic pain. When dealing with a purely female population, a urinary dipstick is likely to be less predictive as a significant proportion of women will be menstruating at any one time. In this situation a catheter sample should be used to minimise false positives. Any inflammatory process close to the ureter may also cause haematuria. This is more likely to occur in women than in men, further undermining the specificity of microscopic haematuria for the diagnosis of renal stones. Ovarian torsion in particular can be difficult to distinguish from renal colic on initial assessment. It is unusual for a urinary tract infection to present with acute pelvic pain in the absence of associated urinary symptoms in non-pregnant women. A negative dipstick for nitrites and leucocytes is a simple and effective way to exclude the possibility of urinary infection when the cause of pelvic pain is uncertain.[12]

Urinary pregnancy testing should be carried out on all women in the reproductive age group presenting with acute pelvic pain. Although rupture of an ectopic pregnancy with a negative pregnancy test has been reported, it is very rare and the index woman usually has a history of a recent positive pregnancy test or presumed miscarriage.[13]

Haematological markers and acute-phase proteins can be used to assess women who have acute pelvic pain. White blood cell count and C-reactive protein (CRP)[14] are the most commonly tested markers. The 'acute phase' is a systemic response to tissue injury, so markers are non-specific and can increase in the presence of infarction or haemorrhage as well as infection. Bear in mind that D-dimers and ferritin are also acute-phase reactants, so have very limited use as diagnostic tests in an acutely unwell patient; a raised D-dimer does not necessarily indicate thrombosis[15] and a raised ferritin may mask iron deficiency.[16]

The use of CRP testing is almost ubiquitous in women presenting with pain and can be a useful indicator of underlying organic pathology rather than 'functional' pain. However, CRP levels start to rise only 6–8 hours after the onset of a pathological event and peak at 24–72 hours. In view of this time-lag, the clinical picture should take precedence: a normal CRP level does not exclude pathology, particularly early in the disease process. Conversely, a woman who is well should not be kept in hospital for unnecessary investigations or observation purely because her CRP level is still rising or has not yet returned to normal.

CRP is raised in 80–90% of women with PID and 63% of those with appendicitis. If both the white blood cell count and CRP are normal, the diagnosis of acute appendicitis is very unlikely.[17] The white blood cell count is raised in approximately 50% of women subsequently diagnosed with ovarian torsion.[4]

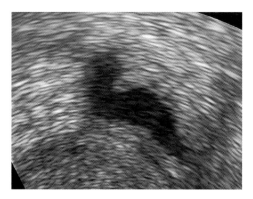

FIGURE 13.5 **Ultrasound image of oedematous thick-walled fallopian tube in acute pelvic inflammatory disease**

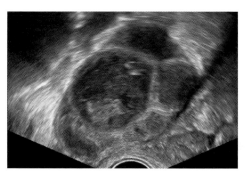

FIGURE 13.6 **Ultrasound image of tubo-ovarian abscess**

Ultrasound

The advantages of ultrasound scanning are that it is safe, accessible and relatively inexpensive. Ultrasound should be used in a dynamic way in the assessment of women in pain. During a gynaecological scan, targeted pressure can be applied gently with the transvaginal probe to help elicit the origin of the pain. The downsides of this technique are that it is operator-dependent and the resolution is best when structures are close to the probe, so the view may be restricted by obesity or fibroids, or if the woman has severe pain.[18]

Normal fallopian tubes are thin and do not contain intraluminal fluid, which makes it difficult to visualise them on ultrasound scan. Acute PID is associated with oedema of the tubal wall and the tube may be dilated with echogenic fluid (pus) (Figure 13.5). Fluid is seen in the pouch of Douglas in 50% of women with PID, but this is a non-specific feature as about one-third of asymptomatic women have free fluid in the pelvis at any time. A tubo-ovarian abscess is seen as a complex, thick-walled multilocular mass in the adnexa that contains echogenic fluid (Figure 13.6). Overall, ultrasound has a relatively low sensitivity for detecting acute PID; however, if characteristic features are seen, they are highly specific.[19] If the clinical diagnosis is clear, imaging is not required. Imaging should be reserved for women who are severely unwell or unresponsive to antibiotics. Ultrasound can then be used to assess whether there is a tubo-ovarian abscess amenable to drainage.

Acute haemorrhagic cysts have a single locule and contain echogenic clots and strands of fibrin. The cyst wall is irregular and well vascularised.[20] There is a clear crescent of normal ovarian tissue surrounding the cyst (Figure 13.7). When pressure is applied with the probe, the clot is seen to be jelly-like and to wobble. Intraperitoneal bleeding from a cyst shows as echogenic fluid, with blood clots surrounding the ovary and in the pouch of Douglas (Figure 13.8).

In ovarian torsion, the ovary is enlarged and oedematous and tends to have peripherally arranged follicles (Figure 13.9). The pedicle that is twisted may be seen as a 'whirlpool'. If there is a simple cyst within the ovary, the cyst tends to become haemorrhagic as the ovary undergoes venous congestion, so the fluid within it becomes more echogenic. The tube may also be involved and may fill with haemorrhagic fluid. The lack of Doppler signals within the ovary may help to confirm the diagnosis, but complete absence of perfusion is a relatively late event, so the presence of flow within the ovary does not exclude the diagnosis of torsion.[4] There is usually haemorrhagic fluid in the pouch of Douglas.

Ovarian hyperstimulation syndrome presents with enlarged ovaries containing multiple luteinised cysts or corpora lutea in association with ascites.

Haematometra can be diagnosed when the uterine cavity is distended with blood (Figure 13.10). If the acute pain is caused by a distended non-communicat-

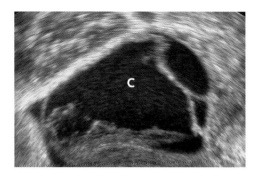

FIGURE 13.7 **Ultrasound image of haemorrhagic ovarian cyst (C)**

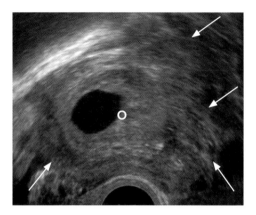

FIGURE 13.8 **Ultrasound image of intraperitoneal bleeding with a blood clot (arrows) surrounding the ovary (O)**

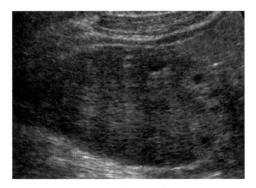

FIGURE 13.9 A **Ultrasound images of ovarian torsion of a polycystic ovary during pregnancy**

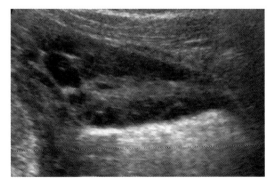

FIGURE 13.9 B **Contralateral ovary appeared polycystic, but with no signs of enlargement or oedema**

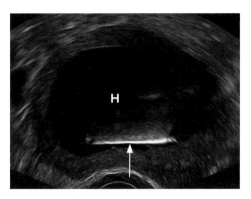

FIGURE 13.10 **Haematometra: a uterine cavity distended by blood (H) with an intrauterine contraceptive device in place (arrow)**

ing rudimentary horn, there will be a vascular pedicle linking it with a unicornuate uterus on the opposite side. If the acute pain is caused by an imperforate hymen, there will be a haematocolpos and the vagina will be filled with fluid. The ultrasound appearance of fibroids does not correlate well with the presence of pain. Most fibroids that on ultrasound have a cystic appearance suspicious of degeneration are entirely painless.[18]

Computed tomography and magnetic resonance imaging

In the UK, computed tomography (CT) and magnetic resonance imaging (MRI) are usually used as second-line tests after ultrasound owing to their lack of availability and their expense. They are not dynamic tests, so do not cause additional discomfort; nor are the images adversely affected by obesity or large fibroids. However, they are also subjective and, similar to ultrasound, the accuracy of the diagnosis is dependent on the ability of the person interpreting the scan.

CT has the disadvantage that it involves significant radiation exposure, so should be avoided in pregnancy where possible. CT is the imaging method of choice for examining the gastrointestinal and urinary tracts, but is less effective in the diagnosis of ovarian pathology, with the exception of dermoid cysts (Figure 13.11). This is because fatty material and teeth within the dermoid can be easily visualised, whereas the fine detail of other types of ovarian cyst tends to be lost.[21]

MRI can be useful for characterising ovarian pathology if the ultrasound diagnosis is unclear. It can occasionally be difficult to distinguish an abscess from an endometrioma on ultrasound; MRI can help to resolve this thanks to the different signal intensities generated by pus and blood. MRI is the investigation of choice for acute abdominal or pelvic pain in pregnancy if ultrasound is negative; the ovaries and

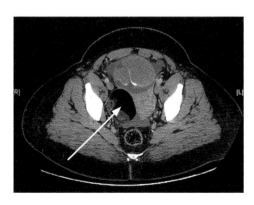

FIGURE 13.11 **Computed tomography image of the pelvis; subcutaneous fat and fat within a dermoid cyst appear black (arrow)**

appendix may be obscured by the gravid uterus or be located too far away from the ultrasound probe to be seen clearly. MRI has a good safety record in pregnancy.[22]

Further investigations and treatment

The treatment of pelvic infection and the role of laparoscopic surgery are covered in other chapters. Haemorrhagic ovarian cysts resolve spontaneously and conservative treatment with analgesia is usually successful. Likewise, haemorrhage from a ruptured functional cyst will usually resolve spontaneously, although women with significant haemoperitoneum should be observed in hospital for 24–48 hours to look for signs of excessive intraperitoneal bleeding and cardiovascular instability.

The most common dilemma is what to do with a woman who complains of persistent pain but in whom all the investigations are negative. Studies have shown that prompt diagnostic laparoscopy reduces the length of hospital stay and facilitates the diagnosis of acute appendicitis. However, only a minority of women who are managed conservatively will require an elective laparoscopy owing to a recurrence of their symptoms over the following year,[23] with the majority of women having pain that resolves spontaneously.[24]

The aims of clinical assessment of women presenting with acute pelvic pain are to provide each individual with a prompt and accurate diagnosis and to initiate appropriate treatment as soon as possible. The longer a woman is in hospital with no resolution of or rational explanation for her symptoms, the sooner she will lose confidence in those caring for her.

Acute pelvic pain can have both gynaecological and non-gynaecological causes, so there will always be a need for collaboration and good communication between different medical specialties when managing women in pain. This will be the case regardless of the variations in the organisation and delivery of emergency gynaecology services in different hospitals. All those caring for acutely ill women should work together in an effort to minimise delays in completing the diagnostic process and starting appropriate management. Provision of out-of-hours imaging and training of gynaecologists in transvaginal ultrasound could help both to establish the cause of pain without delay and to reduce unnecessary admissions to gynaecology wards.

Conclusion

Eliciting a detailed and accurate history gives the most diagnostic information when assessing a woman with acute pelvic pain. Clinical examination, blood tests and imaging can be used to refine the diagnosis so that surgical intervention can be reserved for women needing treatment rather than a diagnosis.

References

1 Morishita K, Gushimiyagi M, Hashiguchi M, Stein G H, Tokuda Y. Clinical prediction rule to distinguish pelvic inflammatory disease from acute appendicitis in women of childbearing age. *Am J Emerg Med* 2007;25:152–7.

2 Centers for Disease Control and Prevention. Sexually Transmitted Diseases: Treatment Guidelines 2006. Pelvic Inflammatory Disease [www.cdc.gov/STD/treatment/2006/pid.htm].

3 Peipert J F, Ness RB, Blume J, Soper DE, Holley R, Randall H, et al.; Pelvic Inflammatory Disease Evaluation and Clinical Health Study Investigators. Clinical predictors of endometritis in women with symptoms and signs of pelvic inflammatory disease. *Am J Obstet Gynecol* 2001;184:856–63.

4 Shadinger L L, Andreotti R F, Kurian R L. Preoperative sonographic and clinical characteristics as predictors of ovarian torsion. *J Ultrasound Med* 2008;27:7–13.

5 Jensen J T, Speroff L. Health benefits of oral contraceptives. *Obstet Gynecol Clin North Am* 2000;27:705–21.

6 James A H. Women and bleeding disorders. *Haemophilia* 2010;16 Suppl 5:160–7.

7 Hibbard L T. Adnexal torsion. *Am J Obstet Gynecol* 1985;152:456–61.

8 Oelsner G, Shashar D. Adnexal torsion. *Clin Obstet Gynecol* 2006;49:459–63.

9 Ahmed Kamel R M. Spontaneous ovarian hyperstimulation syndrome in a naturally conceived singleton pregnancy. *Fertil Steril* 2010;94:351.e1–4.

10 Jayasinghe Y, Rane A, Stalewski H, Grover S. The presentation and early diagnosis of the rudimentary uterine horn. *Obstet Gynecol* 2005;105:1456–67.

11 Bove P, Kaplan D, Dalrymple N, Rosenfield A T, Verga M, Anderson K, et al. Reexamining the value of hematuria testing in patients with acute flank pain. *J Urol* 1999;162:685–7.

12 St John A, Boyd J C, Lowes A J, Price C P. The use of urinary dipstick tests to exclude urinary tract infection: a systematic review of the literature. *Am J Clin Pathol* 2006;126:428–36.

13 Lee J K, Lamaro V P. Ruptured tubal ectopic pregnancy with negative serum beta hCG – a case for ongoing vigilance? *N Z Med J* 2009;122:94–9.

14 Azizia M M, Irvine L M, Coker M, Sanusi F A. The role of C-reactive protein in modern obstetric and gynecological practice. *Acta Obstet Gynecol Scand* 2006;85:394–401.

15 Wells P S. Integrated strategies for the diagnosis of venous thromboembolism. *J Thromb Haemost* 2007;5 Suppl 1:41–50.

16 Northrop-Clewes C A. Interpreting indicators of iron status during an acute phase response – lessons from malaria and human immunodeficiency virus. *Ann Clin Biochem* 2008;45:18–32.

17 Grönroos J M, Grönroos P. A fertile-aged woman with right lower abdominal pain but unelevated leukocyte count and C-reactive protein. Acute appendicitis is very unlikely. *Langenbecks Arch Surg* 1999;384:437–40.

18 Valentin L. Imaging in gynecology. *Best Pract Res Clin Obstet Gynaecol* 2006;20:881–906.

19 Timor-Tritsch I E, Lerner J P, Monteagudo A, Murphy K E, Heller D S. Transvaginal sonographic markers of tubal inflammatory disease. *Ultrasound Obstet Gynecol* 1998;12:56–66.

20 Swire M N, Castro-Aragon I, Levine D. Various sonographic appearances of the hemorrhagic corpus luteum cyst. *Ultrasound Q* 2004;20:45–58.

21 Kalish G M, Patel M D, Gunn M L, Dubinsky T J. Computed tomographic and magnetic resonance features of gynecologic abnormalities in women presenting with acute or chronic abdominal pain. *Ultrasound Q* 2007;23:167–75.

22 Singh A, Danrad R, Hahn P F, Blake M A, Mueller P R, Novelline R A. MR imaging of the acute abdomen and pelvis: acute appendicitis and beyond. *Radiographics* 2007;27: 1419–31.

23 Gaitán H, Angel E, Sánchez J, Gómez I, Sánchez L, Agudelo C. Laparoscopic diagnosis of acute lower abdominal pain in women of reproductive age. *Int J Gynaecol Obstet* 2002;76:149–58.

24 Harris R D, Holtzman S R, Poppe A M. Clinical outcome in female patients with pelvic pain and normal pelvic US findings. *Radiology* 2000;216:440–3.

14 Management of vaginal bleeding in the acute clinical setting

Natalie AM Cooper and T Justin Clark

Introduction

Heavy vaginal bleeding is a common problem, accounting for approximately 70% of referrals to gynaecologists from primary care. Although this condition is usually encountered in an elective outpatient clinic setting, there are occasions when acute bleeding requires emergency hospital admission. Abnormal vaginal bleeding is the second most common reason for presentation to emergency gynaecology units after acute pelvic pain.

This chapter provides a comprehensive overview of non-pregnancy-associated conditions that might present with acute vaginal bleeding. General approaches to management are described, followed by information and advice on managing specific conditions, with key points to be elicited from the history, signs to search for during clinical examination and information on further investigations and treatment. Acute vaginal bleeding can also result from trauma to the genital tract, including trauma arising from sexual assault. Management of such injuries is discussed.

Acute presentation of vaginal bleeding

Abnormally heavy vaginal bleeding is usually uterine in origin (Box 14.1). A thorough clinical history should be taken with particular regard to previous menstrual problems, past investigations and medical or surgical treatment. Women often present with an acute-on-chronic history of heavy vaginal bleeding and may already be taking oral progestogens in a sporadic fashion. Contraceptive history is also relevant as long-acting reversible contraceptives, such as the levonorgestrel-releasing intrauterine system (Mirena®; Bayer Healthcare Pharmaceuticals Inc., Wayne, NJ, USA) or injectable or implanted progestogens, are often associated with breakthrough bleeding in the first few months of use, which can sometimes be heavy. In the case of Mirena, early expulsion, uterine perforation or infection can result in heavy, often painful bleeding within a few days of the device being fitted. Intermittent use or non-

BOX 14.1 **Differential diagnosis of acute uterine bleeding**

- ○ Dysfunctional uterine bleeding
- ○ Fibroids (intracavitary or prolapsed)
- ○ Retained products of conception
- ○ Contraception-related (recent fitting of intrauterine device or commencement of hormonal contraception)
- ○ Trauma
- ○ Acute pelvic infection with endometritis
- ○ Uterine malignancy
- ○ Uterine inversion
- ○ Haematological disorders in adolescents
- ○ Arteriovenous malformation of the uterus

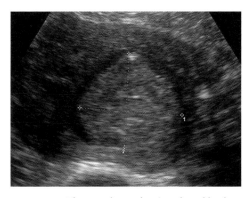

FIGURE 14.1 **Ultrasound scan showing a large blood clot (between calipers) within the uterine cavity in a 48-year-old woman presenting with severely dysfunctional uterine bleeding**

compliance with oral hormonal contraceptives can also lead to unscheduled and heavy bleeds. A sexual history with respect to new sexual partners can also be pertinent, especially in women using intrauterine contraceptive devices. Ascending uterine and pelvic infection can cause acute uterine bleeding, especially if there is a history of pelvic pain and/or vaginal discharge. Pregnancy should always be considered in any woman of reproductive age presenting acutely with abnormal vaginal bleeding.

The most common cause of acute vaginal bleeding in perimenopausal parous women is anovulatory dysfunctional uterine bleeding, which is sometimes compounded by the presence of concomitant uterine pathology. In some cases heavy bleeding can be caused by an acutely prolapsed uterine fibroid that has been expelled through the cervix into the vagina. Young nulliparous women (teenagers or women in their early 20s) can occasionally present with acute bleeding. In these women it is important to consider the diagnosis of underlying coagulopathies such as haemophilia, von Willebrand's disease, platelet aggregation disorders and so on.

Once a detailed history has been obtained, systemic and pelvic examinations should be performed. Vital signs should be recorded, as should any tenderness or presence of abdominopelvic masses. A speculum examination should be performed to assess the amount of bleeding and to exclude cervicitis, cervical polyps, masses or ulcerations or a prolapsed submucous uterine fibroid. A bimanual examination should follow to identify any uterine enlargement suggestive of fibroids or adenomyosis, to assess uterine mobility (a fixed uterus may be caused by adhesions, endometriosis or malignancy) and to check for the presence of any adnexal masses. The internal examination may help to locate areas of tenderness indicative of pelvic infection.

A urinary pregnancy test should be performed in all women of reproductive age, as should a full blood count with or without a group and save, depending on the severity of the bleeding and the haemodynamic state of the woman. A pelvic ultrasound should be performed. This test can provide useful information to aid diagnosis and influence clinical decision making (Box 14.2).

Causes of acute heavy vaginal bleeding and principles of management

Dysfunctional uterine bleeding

The haemodynamic state of the woman should be assessed first and the likely cause of bleeding should be established. A decision should then be made whether acute admission of the patient to hospital is indicated to ensure effective resuscitation and symptom control. The majority of women presenting acutely with heavy vaginal bleeding will be in their fifth decade of life and they usually have a background history of menstrual problems. Women tend to present as emergencies because of severe acute bleeding with passage of large blood clots or because of prolonged, unremitting bleeding. Following a thorough history and pelvic examination, an ultrasound scan should be performed (Figure 14.1). In the absence of any detectable uterine or adnexal abnormalities, the diagnosis of dysfunctional uterine bleeding can be made.

Once significant gynaecological or systemic pathology has been excluded, women who are not cardiovascularly compromised should be discharged home and outpatient follow-up arranged. In the absence of any contraindications, treatment with tranexamic acid (1 g four times daily) should be instigated before discharge. Non-steroidal anti-inflammatory drugs, for example mefenamic acid 500 mg three times daily, can be prescribed to

> **BOX 14.2 Management of women presenting with acute vaginal bleeding**
>
> ○ History
>
> ○ Systemic and pelvic examination
>
> ○ Urinary pregnancy test
>
> ○ Full blood count and blood group and save
>
> ○ Pelvic ultrasound scan
>
> ○ Treat according to diagnosis:
>
> > ▷ Dysfunctional uterine bleeding – tranexamic acid and oral progestogens; consider combined oral contraceptive/ gonadotrophin-releasing hormone analogues (second line)
> >
> > ▷ Prolapsed uterine fibroid – vaginal myomectomy
> >
> > ▷ Arteriovenous malformation – hormonal treatment, arterial embolisation, surgery
> >
> > ▷ Clotting disorder – liaise with haematologist and give factor replacement, desmopressin, tranexamic acid, etc. as appropriate
> >
> > ▷ Endometritis /pelvic inflammatory disease – antibiotics
> >
> > ▷ Uterine malignancy – endometrial sampling and refer to oncologist
> >
> > ▷ Retained products of conception – evacuation of retained products of conception
>
> ○ Admit woman if haemodynamically unstable and/or symptomatic anaemia and resuscitate (intravenous fluids, iron supplementation ± blood transfusion)
>
> ○ Arrange outpatient follow-up (general gynaecology or outpatient hysteroscopy clinic)

women who also complain of painful bleeding. Where bleeding is prolonged and irregular, systemic progestogens can be commenced, such as norethisterone 5 mg three times daily or medroxyprogesterone acetate 10 mg three times daily. The instructions for use and duration of medical treatment should be discussed with the woman and her primary care physician should be informed of the management plan. In general, tranexamic acid is taken until bleeding starts to subside and oral progestogens are given for between 5 and 10 days. Ferrous sulphate should be prescribed if there is evidence of iron-deficiency anaemia.

Women should be admitted to an inpatient ward if home support is lacking and vaginal bleeding is unduly excessive, especially in the presence of severe, symptomatic anaemia, haemodynamic instability or sepsis. A lower threshold for admission should be reserved for women with other medical comorbidities. Medical treatment for heavy bleeding as described above should be commenced. In addition, women should be given intravenous fluids and provided with effective pain control if required. Blood transfusion and/or intravenous iron therapy (iron sucrose or iron dextran) should be considered in the presence of severe iron-deficiency anaemia, especially if the bleeding is slow to cease and the woman is symptomatic or haemodynamically unstable.

Once the acute episode has settled, discharge with outpatient follow-up should be arranged and more definitive, longer-term treatment instituted. In practice, relevant investigations, such as uterine imaging, hysteroscopy and endometrial biopsy, can be completed and a definitive plan of management formulated during the inpatient stay. If a subsequent hysterectomy is planned, the use of gonadotrophin-releasing hormone analogues should be considered, especially in the presence of significant uterine fibroids or iron-deficiency anaemia.

Prolapsed uterine fibroid

Uterine fibroids are a common cause of heavy vaginal bleeding associated with iron-deficiency anaemia. Women with prolapsed fibroids often present acutely, although this is often preceded by a history of chronic heavy menstrual bleeding. Expulsion of a uterine fibroid through the cervix and into the vagina usually occurs spontaneously; however, it has also been described following uterine artery embolisation,[1–5] endometrial ablation[6] and medical treatment of fibroids with gonadotrophin-releasing hormone analogues.[7,8]

The diagnosis of a prolapsed uterine fibroid is usually obvious on speculum examination, which allows visualisation of the protruding fibroid. The lesion may be partially degenerated or necrotic and it may resemble malignant uterine or cervical pathology. Digital exploration is useful to enable examination of the cervix, which may be difficult to see on speculum examination in cases of large prolapsed fibroids. The pedicle with which the fibroid is attached to the uterine cavity is also sometimes easier to locate on palpation. Ultrasound examination may be helpful to visualise the site of pedicle insertion within the uterine cavity and to detect any additional uterine abnormalities (Figures 14.2 and 14.3). Ultrasound examination may also facilitate the rare diagnosis of fibroid-induced uterine inversion (see below).

Treatment of prolapsed uterine fibroids is surgical and involves a vaginal myomectomy (Box 14.3). The procedure can be performed in an outpatient hysteroscopy clinic setting with or without local cervical anaesthesia, but it usually requires general anaesthesia in a formal operating theatre. The authors' preference is to place the patient in the lithotomy position and perform an initial vaginoscopic hysteroscopy to identify the uterine cavity, thus excluding a uterine inversion, and to locate the intrauterine attachment of the fibroid pedicle. The fibroid can then be grasped with one or two toothed forceps, such as a double-toothed vulsellum or a Littlewoods tissue forceps, and avulsed in the same manner used in an open myomectomy. An alternative approach is to put the extruded fibroid under tension with the grasping forceps to identify the attaching pedicle and use hand-held diathermy to excise the fibroid or to ligate the pedicle prior to dividing it. A potential advantage of the latter approach is that some of the feeding myometrial blood vessels will be sealed, thereby reducing the blood loss. However, in clinical practice it is often difficult to obtain good access to the pedicle and to secure it. Very large fibroids should be removed by surgical debulking and piecemeal extraction.

Once the vaginal myomectomy has been completed, the lower genital tract should be observed for signs of bleeding. If bleeding is excessive, a Foley catheter can be inserted into the uterus with the aid of an atraumatic ring sponge forceps. The balloon should be inflated to between 10 and 30 ml to provide temporary tamponade. Uterotonic agents such as ergometrine or prostaglandins such as misoprostol or carboprost should be given. The balloon catheter can usually be safely deflated and removed within 4 hours.

Uterine inversion

Uterine inversion in non-pregnant women is very rare. In the acute gynaecological setting, most cases are associated with fibroids, polyps or uterine malignan-

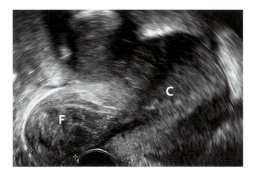

FIGURE 14.2 **Longitudinal view of the uterus showing a large prolapsed submucous fibroid (F) in a woman presenting with a history of acute heavy vaginal bleeding**

C = uterine corpus.

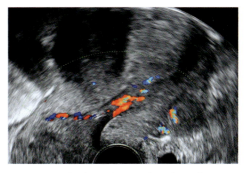

FIGURE 14.3 **The diagnosis is confirmed on colour Doppler showing a thick vascular pedicle connecting the fibroid to the uterine cavity**

BOX 14.3 **Vaginal myomectomy following fibroid expulsion**

- Prescribe antibiotics if the fibroid appears necrotic
- Use the lithotomy position
- Identify the uterus (palpation, ultrasound and/ or hysteroscopy)
- Consider ligation of the fibroid pedicle
- Avulse or excise the vaginal fibroid using traumatic grasping tissue forceps
- Observe for vaginal bleeding
- Intrauterine tamponade (e.g. Foley catheter) if there is continued bleeding ± uterotonic agents

cies,[9–11] but spontaneous, idiopathic inversion can also occur. The mechanism of inversion is unclear; the probable cause is expulsion of the fibroid through the cervix. If the fibroid is attached to the fundal aspect of the cavity by a short pedicle, the expulsion through the cervix exerts a downward traction on the fundus, which can cause inversion. This is similar to iatrogenic inversion, which can occur as a result of manual traction on the fibroid.

Uterine inversion presents in the same way as the more common pro-lapse of a uterine fibroid, with acute or acute-on-chronic bleeding, pelvic pain and, occasionally, haemodynamic shock. A speculum examination will reveal a mass protruding through a dilated cervix. It can be very difficult to distinguish inversion from a prolapsed fibroid, so an ultrasound scan, magnetic resonance imaging[12] or examination under anaesthesia is usually necessary to reach a correct diagnosis. If a 'fibroid' stalk cannot be felt on examination or there is difficulty feeling the uterus, the rare diagnosis of uterine inversion should be considered. An inability to bypass the intravaginal mass to enter and identify the uterine cavity at hysteroscopy also suggests an inversion.

Conservative treatment of uterine inversion is sometimes possible using manual or hydrostatic replacement of the inverted uterus, but recurrent inver-sion can be a problem. Surgical approaches are either abdominal (Haultain and Huntingdon techniques) or vaginal (Kustner and Spinelli techniques)[13] and involve anatomical repositioning by upward traction, with or without incision of the vaginocervical 'ring' created by the inversion. The decision to proceed to hysterectomy should be made depending on the age and haemodynamic state of the woman, whether bleeding is controlled, the likelihood of recurrent inversion and the underlying diagnosis (such as uterine malignancy).

Uterine arteriovenous malformations

Uterine arteriovenous malformations (AVMs) are proliferations of arterial and venous channels with vascular fistula formation. They should be considered in the differential diagnosis of causes of acute vaginal bleeding. Bleeding can be profuse (like 'turning on a tap') and prolonged, often requiring a blood transfu-sion. Uterine AVMs are either congenital or acquired.[14] Congenital AVMs have multiple vascular connections, usually present early (in teenagers and women in their early 20s) and may also be present at extrauterine sites. Acquired AVMs usually have a single connection between an artery and a vein. They may occur after a miscarriage or a molar pregnancy. Acquired AVMs can also develop after surgical operations on the uterus, such as uterine curettage, caesarean section, removal of intrauterine devices and myomectomy (Box 14.4).

The diagnosis of uterine AVMs is usually made on transvaginal ultrasound with the aid of colour Doppler imaging. A uterine AVM will be identified on a grey-scale ultrasound of the pelvis by the presence of small anechoic cystic lesions within the underlying myo-metrium.[15] On colour Doppler examination uterine AVMs demonstrate high vascularity extending towards the subendometrial layer with multidirectional, tur-bulent, low-impedance, high-velocity flow typical of arteriovenous shunting.[16,17] Highly vascular retained products of conception can sometimes be mistaken for an AVM on transvaginal ultrasound (Figures 14.4 and 14.5).[18] Computed tomography and magnetic res-onance imaging may be used to determine the size, extent and vascularity of the AVM and the involvement of adjacent organs.[19] Digital subtraction angiography is considered by some as the gold standard test for detect uterine AVMs; this procedure should be per-formed if ultrasound findings are equivocal.[19] On angi-ography, the common and internal iliac arteries appear thicker and more circuitous on the affected compared with the normal side. AVMs appear as a complex tan-gle of vessels supplied by enlarged feeding arteries.

Treatment of confirmed uterine AVMs can be medical, radiological or surgical. In the past, intracta-ble haemorrhage without an apparent cause required hysterectomy, while uterine AVMs were diagnosed on histopathological examination of the uterus. With the advent of more sophisticated imaging, uterine AVMs can be diagnosed preoperatively and conserva-tive treatment can be used. Traumatic and acquired pregnancy-related uterine AVMs can regress spontane-ously, which justifies an expectant approach in the first instance, especially with a first, self-limiting presenta-tion in a young, haemodynamically stable woman with a desire for future fertility and a small vascular abnor-mality.[17] Medical treatments with prostaglandins, such as 15-methyl-prostaglandin analogues, or sex-steroid hormones have been successfully used. The authors' preference is to suppress the endometrium either with

BOX 14.4 **Clinical presentation suggestive of a uterine arteriovenous malformation**

- Recurrent severe episodes of uterine bleeding with anaemia ± requirement for blood transfusion

- Bleeding refractory to medical and hormonal treatments

- Under 25 years of age

- Past history of uterine surgery/miscarriage

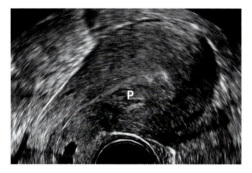

FIGURE 14.4 **Longitudinal view of the uterus showing a small amount of retained products of conception (P)**

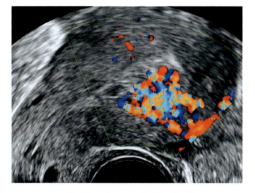

FIGURE 14.5 **On Doppler examination the tissue is highly vascular, resembling an arteriovenous malformation**

Uterine vascularity typically returns to normal following surgical evacuation of retained products.

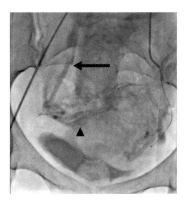

FIGURE 14.6 A **Left internal iliac angiogram showing a vascular 'tangle' supplied by the left uterine artery (arrow)**

Courtesy of Dr Robert Jones.

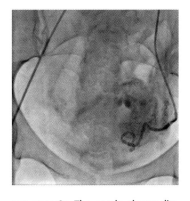

FIGURE 14.6 B **The vascular abnormality is not visible after selective embolisation**

Courtesy of Dr Robert Jones.

high-dose systemic progestins or the combined oral contraceptive pill. Hormonal treatment should be continued in the longer term and regular follow-up arranged to judge symptomatic and radiological response. The acute management of heavy menstrual bleeding associated with an AVM is outlined in Box 14.5.

Targeted uterine artery embolisation is indicated if bleeding persists (usually owing to larger lesions involving subendometrial tissue) to the degree that blood transfusions are required to maintain haemodynamic stability, or in women who have recurrent episodes of bleeding requiring repeated acute hospital admissions (Figures 14.6 A, B). Angiographic arterial embolisation is preferred over surgical interventions as it provides an immediate, minimally invasive and fertility-sparing treatment. Women should be asked to provide consent for this possible intervention prior to the diagnostic arteriogram. Sometimes the procedure has to be repeated to achieve successful resolution of symptoms. The majority of women will revert to a normal menstrual cycle, which may be related to the fact that embolisation is a selective process that blocks the vessels leading to the malformation and spares the ovarian circulation.

Surgical treatments for uterine AVMs include repeated hysteroscopic coagulation of the lesion (although intraoperative bleeding often limits the success of this approach), laparoscopic or open coagulation, clipping or formal ligation of the uterine arteries. Hysterectomy can be used should these approaches fail. It should be noted that uterine curettage is not therapeutic and will generally aggravate bleeding.

Haematological disorders

Women presenting acutely with heavy vaginal bleeding are usually parous and perimenopausal, or have significant uterine fibroids. When adolescent and teenage girls or nulliparous women in their early 20s present as emergencies with heavy vaginal bleeding, haemostatic disorders or uterine vascular anomalies should be considered as possible causes. The prevalence of inherited bleeding disorders in the general population of women with heavy vaginal bleeding is estimated to be between 10% and 20%.[20,21]

Haemostatic abnormalities include platelet dysfunction (platelet function defects, thrombocytopenia), von Willebrand's disease and coagulation factor deficiencies. Von Willebrand's disease – a qualitative or quantitative deficiency of von Willebrand's factor, a multimeric protein required for platelet adhesion – is by far the most common hereditary disorder of coagulation. Its prevalence in women with heavy vaginal bleeding is approximately 13%. These inherited bleeding disorders are found in women of all reproductive ages with heavy vaginal bleeding. The National Institute for Health and Clinical Excellence (NICE), in its guideline on heavy menstrual bleeding, states that 'testing for coagulation disorders should be considered in women who have had heavy periods since menarche and have personal or family history suggesting a coagulation disorder'.[22]

In the majority of teenagers presenting with heavy vaginal bleeding, the diagnosis is one of self-limiting anovulatory dysfunctional uterine bleeding arising from immaturity of the hypothalamic–pituitary–ovarian axis. A family history of bruising and bleeding (epistaxis, sports injuries and haemostatic challenges such as dental extractions or childbirth) is suggestive of an underlying bleeding disorder.[23] Therefore, formal coagulation testing could be restricted to those teenagers presenting with heavy vaginal bleeding and a positive bleeding history, as advocated by NICE.

Teenagers diagnosed with anovulatory dysfunctional uterine bleeding should be reassured that their symptoms are likely to be self-limiting. First-line medical treatments include tranexamic acid with or without the use of a nonsteroidal anti-inflammatory agent such as mefenamic acid. In the absence of contraindications and in the presence of refractory menstrual symptoms, especially where contraception is required, teenagers and young women with heavy vaginal bleeding should be offered the combined oral contraceptive pill. In young women confirmed to have an inherited bleeding disorder, both tranexamic acid and the Mirena intrauterine system have been successfully used to control excessive bleeding.[24–26] Mirena should be used as a second- or third-line treatment option in young nulliparous women as the insertion may require general anaesthesia.

Where menstrual symptoms associated with inherited bleeding disorders are resistant to standard, evidence-based treatment approaches, treatment with 1-desamino-8-d-arginine vasopressin (desmopressin, or DDAVP) either parenterally or via nasal spray should be considered in consultation with a haematologist. DDAVP, a vasopressin analogue, acts on antidiuretic hormone receptors to increase clotting factors (factor VIII) and platelet adherence. However, DDAVP has not been shown to be significantly better than placebo[27] or tranexamic acid[28] for the treatment of heavy vaginal bleeding.

BOX 14.6 **Management of adolescent and young women presenting acutely with heavy menstrual bleeding**

- History
- Systemic and pelvic examination*
- Urinary pregnancy test
- Blood tests
  - Full blood count (haemoglobin and platelet count) ± blood group and save
  - Haemostatic evaluation (coagulation tests – prothrombin time, partial thromboblastin time; von Willebrand's screening – vWf:Ag, vWf:AC and FVIII levels [FVIII:C]; platelet function tests – bleeding time, aggregation and release studies; discuss with laboratory)
- Pelvic ultrasound scan*
- Treat according to diagnosis:
  - Dysfunctional uterine bleeding – tranexamic acid, mefanamic acid ± combined oral contraceptive pill (oral progestogens if there is continuing acute bleeding)
  - Inherited bleeding disorder – liaise with haematologist; standard treatments as above ± desmopressin acetate nasal spray if refractory; specific haematological therapy
  - As described in Box 14.2
- Admit if haemodynamically unstable and/ or symptomatic anaemia and resuscitate (intravenous fluids and iron supplementation, and consider blood transfusion)
- Arrange multidisciplinary outpatient follow-up

*Limit to abdominal examination if the woman is not sexually active.

FVIII factor = VIII | FVIII:C = coagulation factor VIII | vWf:AC = von Willebrand factor activity | vWf:Ag = von Willebrand factor antigen.

The presence of haemostatic abnormalities such as clotting factor deficiency, thrombocytopenia or platelet dysfunction should be managed jointly with a haematologist. This is also true when acute genital tract bleeding is associated with anticoagulation therapy such as warfarin, heparin or antiplatelet drugs, especially if the bleeding time, prothrombin time and/or partial thromboblastin time are markedly prolonged. Systemic illness can also lead to deranged clotting, which usually occurs in older women with chronic illness such as liver or renal disease, so the excessive uterine bleeding should be managed in conjunction with the appropriate medical specialty. Box 14.6 summarises the approach to management of adolescent and young women presenting acutely with heavy menstrual bleeding.

Acute bleeding and use of hormonal contraception

Breakthrough bleeding is common with the combined oral contraceptive pill, but acute presentation with heavy vaginal bleeding is unusual. Unscheduled bleeding with progestogenic contraceptives is also common. Excessive, persistent bleeding is more often seen with the depot preparations such as Depo-Provera® (Pfizer Inc., New York, NY, USA) rather than implants such as Implanon® (Schering-Plough, Kenilworth, NJ, USA). In general, once significant gynaecological pathology is excluded, the best approach is reassurance as symptoms usually settle with the continuation of depot contraception. If treatment is required, tranexamic acid or supplemental estrogen – Premarin® (Wyeth Pharmaceuticals Inc., Philadelphia, PA, USA) 0.625–1.25 mg once daily or a low-dose combined oral contraceptive for 2–3 months – can be administered. The levonorgestrel-releasing intrauterine system Mirena can be associated with persistent acute vaginal bleeding in the first 6 months of use.

Postmenopausal bleeding

Postmenopausal bleeding is a common problem,[29] but the bleeding is rarely so profuse as to warrant acute intervention. However, postmenopausal bleeding is an alarming symptom because of the relatively high risk of endometrial cancer, so women are sometimes referred to accident and emergency departments by their general practitioners. The majority of women with postmenopausal bleeding have benign pathology, such as atrophy of the genital tract, endometrial polyps, submucosal fibroids, endometrial hyperplasia without atypia, endometritis and impaired coagulation.[29] In 10–15% of women with postmenopausal bleeding, endometrial cancer or complex endometrial hyperplasia with cytological atypia will be present. A suggested approach to the on-call management of postmenopausal bleeding is given in Box 14.7.

BOX 14.7 **Acute management of postmenopausal bleeding**

- History – elicit risk factors for serious endometrial pathology, e.g. amount, duration, recurrence, older age, non-use of hormone replacement therapy, tamoxifen therapy, diabetes, obesity and family history

- Examination – assess the lower genital tract to exclude vulval lesions (especially in elderly women), assess the vaginal and cervical pathology and perform smear test if not up to date; exclude bleeding from other sources, e.g. rectum or bladder

- Pelvic ultrasound – perform or arrange promptly a transvaginal scan to assess the endometrial thickness and adnexae ± endometrial biopsy

- Outpatient follow-up – arrange urgent (<2 weeks) outpatient assessment according to local policies (postmenopausal bleeding pathways, oncology clinics)

As a prompt diagnostic work-up is essential, where possible, proactive assessment ('getting the ball rolling') should be encouraged rather than simply arranging scheduled outpatient assessment. However, arranging for referred women to attend a specialist postmenopausal bleeding clinic may be the most efficient and suitable way to investigate their condition, as it will ensure that they are seen quickly and followed up appropriately. A further consideration is that it can be logistically difficult to examine women adequately in a non-gynaecological setting as general wards are not set up for positioning the patient appropriately, nor do they have the necessary equipment or lighting. Ultrasound assessment of double-layer endometrial thickness should be the first-line diagnostic test in postmenopausal bleeding.[30] It may be helpful and efficient to arrange this test in advance of the urgent outpatient appointment (Figures 14.7 and 14.8).

Heavy vaginal bleeding after the menopause leading to severe anaemia and haemodynamic compromise is rare, but when seen is usually caused by an advanced cervical or endometrial cancer. This emergency situation requires immediate resuscitation with administration of oxygen, intravenous fluid replacement and blood transfusion depending on the full blood count and clotting results. A pelvic examination should be performed in an appro-

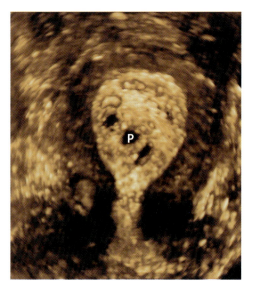

FIGURE 14.7 **Three-dimensional ultrasound scan showing a large cystic benign endometrial polyp (P) in a woman presenting with heavy postmenopausal bleeding**

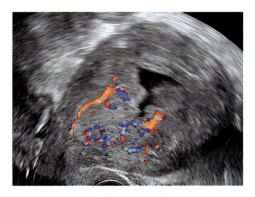

FIGURE 14.8 **Longitudinal section of the uterus showing a large vascular tumour within the uterine cavity in a woman with a history of recurrent heavy postmenopausal bleeding**

These findings are typical of endometrial cancer.

priate setting with adequate lighting, with recourse to examination under general anaesthesia if access and visualisation are suboptimal. Once the source of bleeding is established, attempts should be made to suppress the haemorrhage. If the bleeding is from a friable cervical or vaginal mass that has not previously been noted, it is advisable to obtain a tissue biopsy. An endometrial biopsy should be obtained in women in whom acute bleeding is coming from within the uterus. Antibiotics should be given and swabs taken if the mass is necrotic or appears infected. Vaginal packing can be employed to stop bleeding from the cervix or vagina with or without the additional use of an absorbable surface haemostatic agent such as Surgicel® (Ethiicon, Inc., Somerville, NJ, USA) or Lyostypt® (B Braun Biosurgicals, Tuttlingen, Germany), or a topical thrombin such as FloSeal® haemostatic matrix (Baxter Healthcare Corporation, Fremont, CA, USA). Women presenting acutely in this manner have often been previously diagnosed with uterine or cervical cancer. Whether these women are known to cancer services or not, early liaison with oncologists is recommended for further planning. In the case of unremitting vaginal blood loss, liaison with other medical disciplines is necessary to arrange haemostatic interventions as well as blood and clotting factor replacement (haematology), urgent radiotherapy (medical oncology) or emergency arterial embolisation (interventional radiology). High-dose systemic progestogens such as medroxyprogesterone acetate and the antifibrinolytic tranexamic acid can also be used to suppress acute bleeding of endometrial origin while further management is arranged.

Abnormal bleeding in women on hormone replacement therapy

The approach to the management of women presenting to acute services with unscheduled or heavy uterine bleeding associated with tamoxifen or hormone replacement therapy (HRT) use should be the same as that used for women with postmenopausal bleeding, as described in the preceding section. It is important to check that compliance with HRT, especially the use of progestins, is adequate. In women who have recently commenced HRT and in whom clinical examination is normal, reassurance should be given that the abnormal bleeding should cease given time.[29] In the absence of overt abnormal pathology, options for prompt reduction or cessation of bleeding related to the use of exogenous hormones include stopping HRT, adding supplemental systemic progestins or using the haemostatic agent tranexamic acid. Prompt outpatient follow-up should be arranged to evaluate the endometrium and exclude an underlying treatable benign pathology such as uterine polyps, a hyperplastic process or endometrial malignancy.[29]

Genital tract trauma

Trauma to the genital tract can cause a variety of injuries, including vaginal laceration or tears, vulval haematomas and haematomas at the pouch of Douglas. Mechanisms of genital tract trauma include straddle or crossbar injuries,[31–33] injuries involving jets of water (for example during water- or jet-skiing),[34–37] pelvic fractures and insertion of foreign bodies into the vagina by children or women with psychiatric disorders. Genital tract trauma can occur with consensual[38,39] and non-consensual sexual intercourse.[40] For example, during consensual sexual intercourse trauma may be caused by fingernails or foreign bodies. Postmenopausal women are at risk of tearing during sexual intercourse if the vagina is atrophic and at sexual debut. Over-exuberance can also cause injury. The mechanism of sexual injury is important as there is a risk that the woman has been the victim of a sexual assault. It is important to ask the woman about this when her partner is not present as she may be reluctant to admit an assault in the presence of an abusive partner (see the section below addressing sexual assault, page 195).

Active bleeding arising from genital tract trauma has often stopped by the time the woman arrives at hospital. However, profuse, potentially life-threatening bleeding can occur and the woman may need full resuscitation before her injuries can be assessed. In this situation, vaginal packing should be used, if tolerated by the woman, to tamponade the genital tract before taking the woman to theatre for a thorough examination under general anaesthesia. A full assessment of the injuries can then be made with adequate lighting and access (with the woman in the lithotomy position) and appropriate surgical treatment carried out. In addition to the assessment of lower genital tract injury, the possibility of internal bleeding within the abdominal cavity should not be overlooked. This is particularly important if the woman complains of abdominal pain or shows signs of cardiovascular instability, abdominal

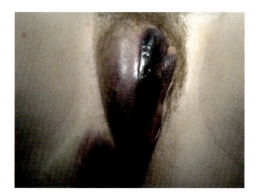

FIGURE 14.9 **Sex-induced vulval haematoma**

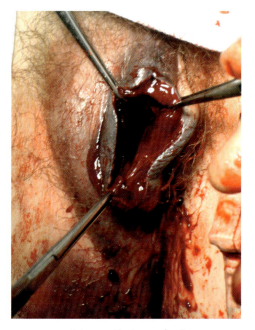

FIGURE 14.10 **Intraoperative image showing evacuation of sex-induced vulval haematoma**

distension and peritoneal irritation. An ultrasound scan should be performed as a minimum to look for internal haemorrhage, with recourse to laparoscopy or indeed laparotomy according to the clinical findings.

More commonly, the presentation is less dramatic. Bleeding has often ceased and the woman is haemodynamically stable and comfortable. External inspection of the vulva and perineum will facilitate detection of any significant vulvovaginal haematomas. These are invariably painful and alarming, so adequate analgesia should be administered, a comfortable bed on the ward provided and transfer to theatre for early surgical drainage expedited. In the absence of a significant vulval haematoma, a gentle speculum examination should be attempted to assess the vagina for lacerations and foreign bodies. Avoid a 'blind' digital examination as sharp foreign bodies such as broken glass may be present. The pouch of Douglas can then be assessed using bimanual examination to feel for any collections. In practice, the examination is often too uncomfortable; if this is the case, an examination under anaesthesia should be arranged. If a small pelvic haematoma is present and the patient is stable, conservative management with the addition of antibiotics to prevent abscess formation is appropriate, after repair of any vaginal lacerations. At examination under anaesthesia, the blood clot should be evacuated and vaginal lacerations should be repaired. Larger haematomas should be incised and evacuated and bleeding points ligated or cauterised if identifiable. Adequate drainage is important if there is continuing 'oozing'; this can be achieved either by de-roofing the haematoma cavity or, preferably, by leaving a drain in place (Figures 14.9 and 14.10). The procedure should be covered with antibiotics to prevent infection and subsequent abscess formation or secondary haemorrhage.

Foreign bodies

Foreign bodies in the vagina can lead to bleeding,[41] infection,[42] lacerations, perforations[43] and fistulae.[44–46] The circumstances surrounding the insertion of foreign bodies are varied. Commonly affected groups of people are psychiatric patients and children, who insert a variety of objects into the vagina (crayons, toys, pens, bottle tops and so on).[41,47] Other common presentations are women who forget to remove tampons, lost condoms, shelf or ring pessaries in older women who have neglected to have them changed and women who have had objects inserted by themselves or by their partners for sexual gratification.[48,49] Occasionally, the object may have been inserted during a sexual assault (see below). In children presenting with offensive vaginal discharge, an undetected foreign body should be suspected. Large, sharp or vigorously inserted objects may cause lacerations or tears and so present more acutely with bleeding and pain.

In cases of suspected foreign body, a full history should be taken and, if possible, details elicited regarding what the object is, how long it has been there and who inserted it. The woman may be reluctant to reveal these details owing to embarrassment, so a sensitive approach is required. The examination should check for haemodynamic compromise caused by bleeding or sepsis. A speculum examination may reveal the foreign body and allow for its removal to be completed in the accident and emergency department or clinic. As mentioned previously, 'blind' digital examination of the genital tract should be avoided unless it is clear from the history that the object is not sharp. Swabs should be taken to check for infections. If the woman is well, she can be discharged with antibiotics if indicated. Patients who are acutely unwell or who cannot tolerate a speculum examination (including children) should be examined and have the foreign body removed under general anaesthesia. Vaginal perforations, lacerations or tears can be repaired at the same time. Examination of the vagina using a hysteroscope is a less invasive method of examining children and virgins and may allow the hymen to be left relatively intact.[50–52] If a fistula is identified, a repair may be scheduled for a later date in consultation with other specialists, such as urologists, colorectal surgeons. Following removal of the foreign body in theatre, women can be discharged home with antibiotic cover. In children, child protection procedures should be implemented if there is any suspicion of abuse.

Sexual assault

If a woman reveals that she has been a victim of a sexual assault, it is vital to make sure she feels safe and has privacy. Avoid leaving the woman on her own for long periods of time. If you are a male doctor, make sure you are accompanied by a female chaperone at all times. If the woman wants to inform the police of the attack, the doctor should make the telephone call.

There is no standardised system across the UK for the management of victims of sexual assault and the approach varies among different regions. If a woman needs to go to theatre, the police may arrange for the forensic doctor to accompany her to theatre to take swabs. This should be discussed with the woman beforehand. Importantly, there are two ways in which you can avoid loss of evidence while waiting for the woman to be assessed by a police doctor. First, keep any sanitary wear that the woman has used, noting whether they were in place during the attack or have been changed since. Second, try to obtain an early evidence kit. If your department does not keep early evidence kits, your accident and emergency department may have one. The kit allows you to take urine and faecal samples and has a mouthwash to allow you to collect samples from the buccal mucosa. This is important if the woman needs to use the toilet or wants to have a drink before she can be examined by the forensic examiner. As well as testing these samples for DNA, the urine sample can be analysed for the presence of drugs. The sooner these samples can be taken, the greater chance there is of collecting important evidence and of finding significant drug levels should they have been a factor in the assault. Ensure that all samples are clearly and correctly labelled.

If the woman does not want to report the attack to the police, you should respect her wishes and maintain confidentiality. However, the woman may change her mind and in these cases your documentation will be crucial. Record as many details as possible using diagrams or photographs taken with a colposcope. Note the position of all injuries, their approximate size, how you repaired them and the estimated blood loss.

As well as treating the injuries caused by a sexual attack, consideration should be given to associated issues. First, address whether the woman needs emergency contraception. Second, consider that the woman may have been exposed to sexually transmitted and blood-borne infections. Chlamydia swabs can be taken during the admission, but you should ensure that the woman has a follow-up appointment arranged with genitourinary medicine services before she is discharged from hospital. Assess whether the woman is at high risk of having been exposed to HIV or hepatitis. A useful website is www.careandevidence.org, which provides clear guidance on how to assess the woman and how to provide postexposure prophylaxis for HIV and vaccines or immunoglobulin for hepatitis B.

Sexual assault is psychological as well as physical. Immediately after an attack, a woman may suffer from rape trauma syndrome, making her unable to remember the details of the attack for 24–48 hours. Later, the woman may develop post-traumatic stress disorder, with flashbacks, intrusive thoughts of the event, nightmares and feelings of confusion, numbness or emptiness. The development of post-traumatic stress disorder is influenced by the woman's situation before the attack and the details of the assault – factors that doctors cannot alter. However, the response of the doctor and how well the woman is supported in the first few days after the attack are also influential and are within the doctor's control. If we show that we believe the woman, take her accusations seriously and keep her safe, we may be able to protect her from long-term suffering caused by the attack. Offer counselling and ensure that the woman is being discharged with a support network in place. Organisations such as rape crisis (www.rape-crisis.org.uk) offer support and counselling for victims of rape and sexual assault.

Child protection procedures should be followed in cases of suspected or confirmed sexual assault of a minor.

A summary of the approach to the acute management of genital tract trauma resulting from sexual assault is described in Box 14.8.

Conclusion

This chapter is essential reading for trainees in acute gynaecology because acute genital tract bleeding accounts for 10–20% of acute gynaecological admissions, coming second only to pelvic pain. The differential diagnoses are numerous and it may be difficult to come to a conclusion on how best to manage women with these conditions. This chapter has covered a wide range of topics, including heavy menstrual bleeding and its associated causes (prolapsed fibroids, AVMs, and so on), bleeding caused by hormonal medications, infections and foreign bodies, gynaecological cancers and trauma and assault. We have provided an overview and advice on the management of each condition with the aim of highlighting important factors in the history and examination that can guide you towards sensible diagnoses and help you to plan the management of the women under your care.

BOX 14.8 **Management of genital tract trauma arising from sexual assault**

- Ensure that the woman feels safe and has privacy.
- Male doctors should be accompanied by a female chaperone at all times.
- Take a history and ensure that the woman understands that you believe her.
- Discuss reporting the attack to the police and respect the woman's decision.
- Follow local procedures for managing victims of sexual assault.
- Use an early evidence kit to take urine and faecal samples and use the mouthwash to collect samples from the buccal mucosa if the woman needs to use the toilet or wants to have a drink before she can be examined by the forensic examiner.
- Examination under general anaesthesia is less traumatising for the woman if injuries need to be explored and repaired.
- Take swabs – this may be performed by a forensic examiner.
- Ensure that samples are correctly labelled and that all documentation is comprehensive. Use diagrams and photographs when possible.
- Discuss antibiotic prophylaxis, postexposure prophylaxis and hepatitis B vaccination.
- Offer emergency contraception.
- Offer counselling and put the woman in touch with support organisations.
- If you suspect sexual assault of a minor, start child protection procedures.

References

1 Murgo S, Simon P, Golzarian J. [Embolization of uterine fibroids]. *Rev Med Brux* 2002;23:435–42. Article in French.

2 Vural B, Ozkan S, Ciftçi E, Bodur H, Yücesoy I. Spontaneous vaginal expulsion of an infected necrotic cervical fibroid through a cervical fistula after uterine artery embolization: a case report. *J Reprod Med* 2007;52:563–6.

3 Radeleff B A, Satzl S, Eiers M, Fechtner K, Hakim A, Rimbach S, et al. [Clinical 3-year follow-up of uterine fibroid embolization]. *Rofo* 2007;179:593–600.

4 Hehenkamp W J, Volkers N A, Van Swijndregt A D, De Blok S, Reekers J A, Ankum W M. Myoma expulsion after uterine artery embolization: complication or cure? *Am J Obstet Gynecol* 2004;191:1713–15.

5 Berkowitz R P, Hutchins F L Jr, Worthington-Kirsch R L. Vaginal expulsion of submucosal fibroids after uterine artery embolization. A report of three cases. *J Reprod Med* 1999;44:373–6.

6 van Riemsdijk V M, Graziosi G C, Veersema S, Bongers M Y. Vaginal myoma expulsion after NovaSure endometrial ablation. *J Minim Invasive Gynecol* 2009;16:496–7.

7 Wen L, Tseng J Y, Wang P H, Vaginal expulsion of a submucosal myoma during treatment with long-acting gonadotropin-releasing hormone agonist. *Taiwan J Obstet Gynecol* 2006;45:173–5.

8 Yu K J, Lai C R, Sheu M H. Spontaneous expulsion of a uterine submucosal leiomyoma after administration of a gonadotropin-releasing hormone agonist. *Eur J Obstet Gynecol Reprod Biol* 2001;96:223–5.

9 Rocconi R, Huh W K, Chiang S. Postmenopausal uterine inversion associated with endometrial polyps. *Obstet Gynecol* 2003;102:521–3.

10 Sharma J B, Kumar S, Rahman S M, Roy K K, Malhotra N. Non-puerperal incomplete uterine inversion due to large sub-mucous fundal fibroid found at hysterectomy: a report of two cases. *Arch Gynecol Obstet* 2009;279:565–7.

11 Mechery J, Crosbie E J, Desai S, Mamtora H, Slade R J. Uterine sarcoma: a rare cause of uterine inversion. *J Obstet Gynaecol* 2009;29:776–8.

12 Lewin J S, Bryan P J. M R imaging of uterine inversion. *J Comput Assist Tomogr* 1989;13:357–9.

13 Buyukkurt S, Vardar M A, Zeren H, Ozgunen F T. Non-puerperal inversion of the uterus caused by leiomyosarcoma: a case report and clinical management. *J Obstet Gynaecol Res* 2007;33:402–6.

14 Fleming H, Ostör A G, Pickel H, Fortune D W. Arteriovenous malformations of the uterus. *Obstet Gynecol* 1989;73:209–14.

15 Torres W E, Sones P J Jr, Thames F M. Ultrasound appearance of a pelvic arteriovenous malformation. *J Clin Ultrasound* 1979;7:383–5.

16 Polat P, Suma S, Kantarcy M, Alper F, Levent A. Color Doppler US in the evaluation of uterine vascular abnormalities. *Radiographics* 2002;22:47–53.

17 Timmerman D, Van den Bosch T, Peeraer K, Debrouwere E, Van S D, Stockx L, et al. Vascular malformations in the uterus: ultrasonographic diagnosis and conservative management. *Eur J Obstet Gynecol Reprod Biol* 2000;92:171–8.

18 Müngen E. Vascular abnormalities of the uterus: have we recently over-diagnosed them? *Ultrasound Obstet Gynecol* 2003;21:529–31.

19 Grivell R M, Reid K M, Mellor A. Uterine arteriovenous malformations: a review of the current literature. *Obstet Gynecol Surv* 2005;60:761–7.

20 James A H, Kouides P A, Abdul-Kadir R, Edlund M, Federici A B, Halimeh S, et al. Von Willebrand disease and other bleeding disorders in women: consensus on diagnosis and management from an international expert panel. *Am J Obstet Gynecol* 2009;201:12.e1–8.

21 El-Hemaidi I, Gharaibeh A, Shehata H. Menorrhagia and bleeding disorders. *Curr Opin Obstet Gynecol* 2007;19:513–20.

22 National Collaborating Centre for Women's and Children's Health. *Heavy menstrual bleeding*. London: RCOG Press; 2007 [nice.org.uk/guidance/CG44].

23 Hayward C P. Diagnosis and management of mild bleeding disorders. *Hematology Am Soc Hematol Educ Program* 2005;423–8.

24 Demers C, Derzko C, David M, Douglas J; Society of Obstetricians and Gynaecologists of Canada. Gynaecological and obstetric management of women with inherited bleeding disorders. *Int J Gynaecol Obstet* 2006;95:75–87.

25 James A H. Von Willebrand disease. *Obstet Gynecol Surv* 2006;61:136–45.

26 Kingman C E, Kadir R A, Lee C A, Economides D L. The use of levonorgestrel-releasing intrauterine system for treatment of menorrhagia in women with inherited bleeding disorders. *BJOG* 2004;111:1425–8.

27 Kadir R A, Lee C A, Sabin C A, Pollard D, Economides D L. DDAVP nasal spray for treatment of menorrhagia in women with inherited bleeding disorders: a randomized placebo-controlled crossover study. *Haemophilia* 2002;8:787–93.

28 Kouides P A, Byams V R, Philipp C S, Stein S F, Heit J A, Lukes A S, et al. Multisite management study of menorrhagia with abnormal laboratory haemostasis: a prospective crossover study of intranasal desmopressin and oral tranexamic acid. *Br J Haematol* 2009;145:212–20.

29 Clark T J, Gupta J K. *Handbook of Outpatient Hysteroscopy. A complete guide to diagnosis and therapy.* London: Hodder Education; 2005.

30 Clark T J, Barton P M, Coomarasamy A, Gupta J K, Khan KS. Investigating postmenopausal bleeding for endometrial cancer: cost-effectiveness of initial diagnostic strategies. *BJOG* 2006;113:502–10.

31 Propst A M, Thorp J M Jr. Traumatic vulvar hematomas: conservative versus surgical management. *South Med J* 1998;91:144–6.

32 Sherer D M, Stimphil R, Hellmann M, Abdelmalek E, Zinn H, Abulafia O. Transperineal sonography of a large vulvar hematoma following blunt perineal trauma. *J Clin Ultrasound* 2006;34:309–12.

33 Virgili A, Bianchi A, Mollica G, Corazza M. Serious hematoma of the vulva from a bicycle accident. A case report. *J Reprod Med* 2000;45:662–4.

34 Haefner H K, Andersen H F, Johnson M P. Vaginal laceration following a jet-ski accident. *Obstet Gynecol* 1991;78:986–8.

35 Kizer K W. Medical hazards of the water skiing douche. *Ann Emerg Med* 1980;9:268–9.

36 Lacy J, Brennand E, Ornstein M, Allen L. Vaginal laceration from a high-pressure water jet in a prepubescent girl. *Pediatr Emerg Care* 2007;23:112–14.

37 Niv J, Lessing J B, Hartuv J, Peyser M R. Vaginal injury resulting from sliding down a water chute. *Am J Obstet Gynecol* 1992;166:930–1.

38 Hoffman R J, Ganti S. Vaginal laceration and perforation resulting from first coitus. *Pediatr Emerg Care* 2001;17:113–14.

39 Jeng C J, Wang L R. Vaginal laceration and hemorrhagic shock during consensual sexual intercourse. *J Sex Marital Ther* 2007;33:249–53.

40 Vermesh M, Deppe G, Zbella E. Non-puerperal traumatic vulvar hematoma. *Int J Gynaecol Obstet* 1984;22:217–19.

41 Stricker T, Navratil F, Sennhauser F H. Vaginal foreign bodies. *J Paediatr Child Health* 2004;40:205–7.

42 Möbus V J, Runnebaum J, Kieback D G, Kreienberg R. [An unusual case: vaginal foreign body (forceps) as an incidental finding during primary operation for breast cancer]. *Geburtshilfe Frauenheilkd* 1995;55:233–4. Article in German.

43 O'Hanlan K A, Westphal L M. First report of a vaginal foreign body perforating into the retroperitoneum. *Am J Obstet Gynecol* 1995;173:962–4.

44 Grody M H, Nyirjesy P, Chatwani A. Intravesical foreign body and vesicovaginal fistula: a rare complication of a neglected pessary. *Int J Urogynecol J Pelvic Floor Dysfunct* 1999;10:407–8.

45 Hirai K, Kita K, Mikata K, Fujikawa N, Kitami K. [Vesicovaginal fistula associated with a vaginal foreign body: a case report]. *Hinyokika Kiyo* 2005;51:283–6. Article in Japanese.

46 Siddiqui N Y, Paraiso M F. Vesicovaginal fistula due to an unreported foreign body in an adolescent. *J Pediatr Adolesc Gynecol* 2007;20:253–5.

47 Stumpf P G. Stenosis and fistulae with neglected vaginal foreign bodies. A case report. *J Reprod Med* 1985;30:559–60.

48 Jaluvka V, Novak A. Vaginal foreign bodies in women in postmenopause and in senium. *Eur J Obstet Gynecol Reprod Biol* 1995;61:167–9.

49 Ahmad M. Intravaginal vibrator of long duration. *Eur J Emerg Med* 2002;9:61–2.

50 Küçük T. When virginity does matter: rigid hysteroscopy for diagnostic and operative vaginoscopy – a series of 26 cases. *J Minim Invasive Gynecol* 2007;14:651–3.

51 Golan A, Lurie S, Sagiv R, Glezerman M. Continuous-flow vaginoscopy in children and adolescents. *J Am Assoc Gynecol Laparosc* 2000;7:526–8.

52 Shui L T, Lee C L, Yen C F, Wang C J, Soong Y K. Vaginoscopy using hysteroscope for diagnosis of vaginal bleeding during childhood: case report. *Changgeng Yi Xue Za Zhi* 1999;22:344–7.

15

Current concepts in screening and outpatient management of pelvic inflammatory disease

Jennifer Hopwood

Introduction

Pelvic inflammatory disease (PID) is an upper genital tract condition. It can be considered as either primary, when there is no obvious contributory factor, or secondary, following an event such as uterine instrumentation with transmission of either an existing infection or commensal bacteria.

Aetiology

There are several organisms that can cause PID: *Chlamydia trachomatis* (5–75%), *Neisseria gonorrhoeae* (5–45%), *Actinomyces*-like organisms (fewer than one in 3000 cases), mycoplasmas/ureaplasmas and, rarely, other bacteria such as *Mycobacterium tuberculosis*[1] and *Salmonella* species. Simms et al.[2] concluded that a high proportion of PID cases are idiopathic, that up to 70% had unidentified aetiology and that behavioural change is a key factor in the primary prevention of PID.

Factors increasing the risk of PID include:

- non-use of condoms

- history of sexually transmitted infections

- uterine instrumentation:
  - insertion of an intrauterine device or intrauterine system if there is a pre-existing infection, or in the first 20 days after insertion[3]
  - hysteroscopy, hysterosalpingography, in vitro fertilisation, surgical termination of pregnancy.

The risk can be reduced by regular use of condoms and spermicides. Contraceptive methods delivering continuous progestogens have the potential to reduce the risk of PID by thickening the cervical mucus; examples include the combined oral contraceptive pill, the progestogen-only pill, Depo-Provera® (Pfizer Inc., New York, NY, USA), Implanon® (Schering-Plough, Kenilworth, NJ, USA) and the Mirena® (Bayer Healthcare Pharmaceuticals Inc., Wayne, NJ, USA) intrauterine system.

Diagnosis

PID accounts for one in 60 GP consultations in women under 45 years of age. The diagnosis is notoriously difficult. The positive predictive value of a clinical diagnosis is 65–90% compared with laparoscopic diagnosis. When evaluating literature on the subject, it is important to be aware that clinical criteria in the studies are likely to differ. Women who are investigated by laparoscopy are likely to have presented with more severe disease than those who receive outpatient treatment.

Women with PID often have malaise, nausea and vomiting. The majority present with lower abdominal pain. In women with Fitz-Hugh–Curtis syndrome, right upper quadrant pain will also be present. Gynaecological symptoms include abnormal vaginal discharge, irregular bleeding and dyspareunia. There may be pyrexia with temperatures above 38°C.

On abdominal palpation there are signs of peritoneal irritation. On pelvic examination there is pain on movement of the cervix ('cervical excitation'). Speculum examination may show offensive vaginal discharge and the cervix often looks inflamed.

Laboratory tests may reveal raised C-reactive protein, erythrocyte sedimentation rate and/or leucocytosis. Microbiological investigation may detect chlamydial or gonococcal infection. The samples used may be first-catch urine, self-taken vulvovaginal swabs or vaginal or endocervical swabs (seek local information about the availability and performance of samples and tests). A pregnancy test should always be performed to exclude early pregnancy complications mimicking PID.

An ultrasound scan should be arranged. This can reveal signs of pyosalpinx or tubo-ovarian abscesses. Free fluid in the lesser pelvis is usually increased in women with acute PID. In women with atypical presentation and inconclusive ultrasound findings, laparoscopy may be necessary to clarify the diagnosis.

The differential diagnosis of PID includes other inflammatory conditions in the abdomen such as appendicitis, diverticulitis and mesenteric adenitis. Gynaecological conditions that could present with similar symptoms to acute PID are endometriosis and ovarian cyst rupture or torsion. Ectopic pregnancy can sometimes be confused with PID.

Management

Mild to moderate PID can be managed on an outpatient basis. The PID Evaluation And Clinical Health (PEACH) study in the USA[4] compared the results of inpatient and outpatient management. The antibiotic treatment used was cefoxitin followed by doxycycline. The conclusion was that 'among women with mild to moderate pelvic inflammatory disease, there was no difference in reproductive outcomes between women randomised to inpatient treatment and those randomised to outpatient treatment'.

There is a general consensus that prompt treatment with antibiotics reduces the risk of long-term adverse sequelae, so there is a low threshold for empirical treatment. Antibiotics should be prescribed to cover *N. gonorrhoea*, *C. trachomatis* and the range of aerobic and anaerobic bacteria that can cause PID. The choice of antibiotics is influenced by the severity of disease, the woman's compliance to treatment (particularly difficult with metronidazole), gonococcal resistance and cost. UK treatment guidelines are provided by the British Association for Sexual Health and HIV[5] and European guidelines by the International Union against Sexually Transmitted Infections.[6]

Antimicrobial therapy

The first-line treatment for PID is ofloxacin 400 mg orally twice daily with metronidazole 400 mg orally twice daily, which should be given for 14 days.

Ofloxacin carries a risk of convulsions in women taking non-steroidal anti-inflammatory drugs. Excessive sunlight should be avoided. Tendon damage including rupture has been reported in patients receiving quinolones.[5,7] Women prescribed antibiotics should be advised of the potential for reduced efficacy of combined oral contraception.

If there is a possibility of pregnancy, erythromycin 500 mg orally twice daily should be used instead of ofloxacin. However, erythromycin is often not well tolerated.

If there is a high risk of gonococcal infection, ofloxacin should be avoided because of increasing resistance to quinolones. This should be considered if the woman's partner is known to have gonorrhoea or her symptoms follow casual sex abroad.

During treatment, women should be advised to take plenty of rest and prescribed adequate analgesia. For women with an intrauterine device or intrauterine system in place, removal should be considered. The current risk and need for emergency contraception, the continuing risk of unwanted pregnancy and the acceptability of alternative methods of contraception should all be considered in the joint decision-making process about whether the intrauterine device or intrauterine system should be removed.

Women treated for PID should be followed up 3 days later to assess the response to treatment, with another review after 1 month. The woman's partner(s) should also be invited for screening and treatment. Women should be advised against intercourse until their partner(s) have been fully investigated and treated if necessary.

Women with severe infections should be admitted and treated with ceftriaxone 250 mg intramuscularly or cefoxitin 2 g intramuscularly with probenecid 1 g orally (not effective for mycoplasmas), followed by doxycycline 100 mg orally twice daily and metronidazole 400 mg orally twice daily for 14 days.

If a diagnosis of PID is made, the woman's partner(s) must be offered empirical treatment as soon as possible. The partner(s) should also have a test for chlamydia and gonorrhoea; if the results are positive, further partner notification will need to be carried out. This may be best effected by a local genitourinary department or a chlamydia clinic, depending on local arrangements. Defined pathways and protocols should be in place.

Women who are HIV-positive should be prescribed the same antibiotics as those listed above, although their symptoms may be more severe than those seen in women without HIV infection.

Women should be advised that fertility is usually preserved if treatment is given promptly. The risk of infertility approximately doubles with each episode of infection and the risk of infertility is greater if the infection is more severe. Chronic pain of varying severity affects 30% of women following an episode of PID. The risk of future pregnancy being ectopic is increased. Additional information for women is available from the RCOG.[8]

Actinomyces-like organisms

Pelvic infection with Actinomyces-like organisms should be considered in women with unresolving PID. Actinomycosis can sometimes cause pelvic and hepatic abscesses. It is an indolent infection requiring a long course of appropriate antimicrobials such as penicillin and metronidazole.

Actinomyces-like organisms can be detected on cervical smears of women using intrauterine devices, but policies are such that many laboratories no longer report their presence. Actinomyces-like organisms are commensals, which usually cause no harm. If they are reported on a cervical smear, the advice of the Clinical Effectiveness Unit of the Faculty of Sexual & Reproductive Healthcare[3] is to establish whether the woman has any symptoms suggestive of clinically relevant infection such as pain or vaginal discharge. If the woman is asymptomatic, the intrauterine device or intrauterine system can be left in place.

Screening to prevent PID

Chlamydia trachomatis

Many publications describing the clinical significance of genital infection with *C. trachomatis* start with the following statement: 'Chlamydia causes pelvic inflammatory disease, which can lead to tubal factor infertility, ectopic pregnancy and chronic pelvic pain'. The extent to which these problems are caused by chlamydial infection remains uncertain. Chlamydia infection may increase the risk of transmission and acquisition of HIV. There are also suggestions that it may be associated with cervical and ovarian cancer. Chlamydia is the most common cause of epididymitis in men under 35 years of age. It also affects babies, causing pneumonitis and conjunctivitis.

Although there is a degree of uncertainty regarding the extent of the long-term effects of chlamydial infection, its short-term morbidity is well documented. In women it can cause urethritis, cervicitis, endometritis, salpingitis and perihepatitis (Fitz-Hugh–Curtis syndrome), so although 70% of infected women are asymptomatic or have only minimal symptoms, some will present with vaginal discharge, dysuria, abnormal bleeding or pelvic pain. Women presenting with any of these symptoms should be offered screening for chlamydia in primary care, as a positive result may avoid the need for referral for a gynaecological or surgical opinion and unnecessary investigations such as laparoscopy, hysteroscopy or colposcopy.

Cervicitis and endometritis can lead to discharge and irregular and post-coital bleeding. Salpingitis causes pelvic pain that may be difficult to differentiate from acute appendicitis or irritable bowel syndrome. Perihepatitis may resemble cholecystitis, while urethritis sometimes mimics cystitis or irritable bladder syndrome. Sexually acquired reactive arthritis can also occur, affecting joints, tendons and skin. Women presenting with any of these symptoms should be screened for chlamydia in primary care before being referred for a gynaecological or surgical opinion. This reduces the risk of women undergoing unnecessary investigations such as laparoscopy, hysteroscopy or colposcopy when the cause of the symptoms is infection rather than other pathology.

However, because the infection is often asymptomatic, the National Chlamydia Screening Programme was rolled out in England in 2007 following a pilot phase. The aim of the programme is 'to control chlamydia through the early detection of asymptomatic infection and reduction of onward disease transmission'.[9] The programme is dependent on good commissioning. It is target-driven, aiming for a sustained target population coverage of 30–50% and robust partner management. Screening is offered opportunistically to women and men under 25 years of age attending general practice, contraception and sexual health clinics. Screening is also offered at other venues such as colleges and prisons and at special events, for example in schools or sports venues. Screening is repeated annually or after a change of partner. The question 'Are you up to date with your chlamydia tests?' can be the norm in a consultation rather than going into a detailed sexual history. The aim of this approach is to destigmatise the infection and increase uptake of screening.

Testing for chlamydia

A portion of the life cycle of chlamydia is intracellular as it requires host cell adenosine triphosphate for energy, so in the past a sample of endothelial cells was required when culture or an enzyme-linked immunosorbent assay was used to test for chlamydia. This meant that invasive samples were needed, which had to be obtained via speculum examination in women or on urethral swabs in men. The introduction of nucleic acid amplification tests (NAATs) for chlamydia detection has led to more ready acceptance of testing among both patients and health professionals. NAATs amplify the chlamydia antigen millions of times so only a small amount is required, such as in a first-catch urine sample or self-taken vulvovaginal swab. Not only is this less intimidating for men and women, but also there are reduced demands on clinical time and therefore costs.

Some NAATs can be used to test for gonorrhoea on the same sample. NAATs include polymerase chain reaction, strand displacement assay and transcription-mediated assay.

The current model for the screening programme is based on evidence that tests were being inconsistently offered in different settings and depended on the degree of interest, time, expertise and funding of a service.[10,11] It was found that, even if a chlamydia test was taken, there were variations in the management of women, often with poor contact tracing.[12,13] This disparity led to the concept of 'chlamydia offices' where all results from all services in a particular area could be consistently managed. A typical office is responsible for supplies to all services in an area: swabs, urine pipetting kits, request forms and publicity and educational material. Chlamydia offices also arrange partner notification and treatment and provide locally and nationally required data. 'You do the test, we do the rest' is the principle behind the model.

Wilson-Jungers criteria for appraising screening programmes have been developed by the National Screening Committee, taking into account international work.[14] Very broadly, the parameters for a screening programme include the following:

- the condition being screened for is an important health problem (both numerically and in terms of severity)

- the natural history of the condition is understood

- there is a suitable, precise and validated test

- there is a process for managing people who test positive on screening and an effective treatment is available

- the cost balance is acceptable

- there are more benefits than risks.

Chlamydia screening measures up against these criteria as follows:

- Is it common? More than 10% of young people tested are positive.

- Is it serious? The sequelae are serious.

- Is the natural history understood? The evidence is far from robust. Probably more than 50% of infections resolve within 1 year, but the factors that contribute to this are not known. The figures relating to the sequelae of chlamydia are based on older studies.

- Is there a test? NAATs fulfil this criterion.

- Is an effective treatment available? Uncomplicated chlamydial infection can be treated with azithromycin 1 g orally immediately or doxycycline 100 mg orally twice daily for 7 days, or erythromycin if the woman is pregnant. The woman's partner(s) should also be tested and treated if necessary.

- What is the balance of risks and benefits? A positive test result can strain or break up relationships and even risk domestic violence. It can also engender considerable worry about future fertility.

Evaluating the evidence

What exactly is the evidence for the extent of the adverse outcomes of chlamydial infection?

Statements such as 'one-third of infertility is tubal factor infertility' and '10% of those with chlamydial infection will develop tubal factor infertility' are based on historical evidence, while statements such as 'chlamydia is an important cause of PID' are based on a large PID study in Sweden in the 1970s.

There are two published randomised controlled trials of chlamydia screening.[15] Women registered in a healthcare setting underwent a single round of testing. PID decreased but there was no observable impact on the prevalence of the infection. The rates of ectopic pregnancies and tubal factor infertility were not assessed. It is difficult to envisage further randomised controlled trials of screening as they would be expensive and require a massive study population with a long follow-up. There is already a high prevalence of chlamydia with a perceived need for action. It should be noted that the action taken differs in different countries, even when using the same evidence.[16]

The argument against screening programmes is based on the uncertain natural history of the infection and statements such as 'The present chlamydia control activities in Sweden, despite being the most extensive in the world, must be regarded as a failure'.[15] There are additional uncertainties related to estimates of coverage requirements, which are calculated to be 30–50% of the target population with good partner notification.[17,18] A further problem for rationalisation of a programme is that one in five people are reinfected at 6 months.

Therefore, there is much more to discover about chlamydia and PID. Gynaecology services often deal with the complications of chlamydia and PID, so they could reasonably and effectively be involved in the evaluation of prevention strategies. In particular, they might be able to contribute to a way of measuring screening success. Large sums of money are invested in screening but there is no measure of outcomes, so it is not possible to work out the cost-effectiveness of screening programmes.

Possible measures of success of a programme in the community include target achievement, number of index cases and partners treated, and reduction in prevalence.

The sequelae of PID, tubal factor infertility and ectopic pregnancies should be expected to reduce over time. The problems involved in studying this are considerable. For example, with PID the diagnosis is inaccurate, some 50% of cases are asymptomatic and 90% of cases occur in the community. With tubal factor infertility, there is the time delay in presentation, the different causes and the fact that not all women present to services – and when they do, they do not necessarily present to the NHS. In addition, when considering the use of serology to establish whether there has been previous chlamydial infection, it must be borne in mind that serological tests need to be species-specific, otherwise a positive result might reflect *C. pneumoniae* rather than *C. trachomatis*.

Examination of ectopic pregnancies has greater potential as a marker of screening success. Sentinel early pregnancy units could be used in conjunction with the screening programme to ascertain whether women with ectopic pregnancies have been previously tested for chlamydial infection and whether they and their partners have been treated, and to establish a decrease over time. It has been found that there is often only a short interval between the chlamydial infection and the ectopic pregnancy.[19] In 20–24-year-old women there is a correlation between chlamydial infection and ectopic pregnancy in the first year, in 20–29-year-old and 30–34-year-old women the chlamydial infection occurs 1 year before the ectopic pregnancy and in 35–39-year-olds the infection occurs 2 years before the ectopic pregnancy.

In areas where a chlamydia screening programme is functioning, it would be expected that women with ectopic pregnancy would have had a previous test. However, on Wirral we have found that, despite 10 years of screening, 75% of women with ectopic pregnancies have not been screened. In addition, we found that although some women with ectopic pregnancies had been tested and treated, their partners had not attended despite all efforts. As with any screening programme, achieving test targets does not reflect the fact that hard-to-reach and vulnerable people may remain untested and, even if they do test positive, will delay accessing treatment.

Conclusion

Tackling chlamydial infection is a cross-specialty issue in which prevention is key. A diagnosis of chlamydia and/or PID requires that the woman's partner(s) are tested and treated too. Current questions about the value of a screening programme should not discourage clinicians from offering the test at every available opportunity, using a local programme infrastructure to optimise care. It is important to provide accurate information about chlamydia in relation to screening programmes, providing reassurance that there is a lower risk of complications than previously thought and stressing that the tests are for genital tract chlamydia, not for PID and its sequelae.

References

1 Aliyu M H, Aliyu S H, Salihu H M. Female genital tuberculosis: a global review. *Int J Fertil Womens Med* 2004;49:123–36.

2 Simms I, Stephenson J M, Mallinson H. Risk factors associated with pelvic inflammatory disease. *Sex Transm Infect* 2006;82:267–75.

3 Faculty of Sexual & Reproductive Healthcare Clinical Effectiveness Unit. *Clinical Guidance: Intrauterine Contraception.* London: Faculty of Sexual & Reproductive Healthcare; 2007 [http://www.ffprhc.org.uk/admin/uploads/ CEUGuidanceIntrauterineCONTRACEPTIONNov07.pdf].

4 Ness R B, Soper D E, Holley R L, Peipert J, Randall H, Sweet R L, et al. Effectiveness of inpatient and outpatient treatment strategies for women with pelvic inflammatory disease: results from the Pelvic Inflammatory Disease Evaluation and Clinical Health (PEACH) randomized trial. *Am J Obstet Gynecol* 2002;186:929–37.

5 British Association for Sexual Health and HIV. *United Kingdom National Guideline for the Management of Pelvic Inflammatory Disease.* London: British Association for Sexual Health and HIV; 2005 [www.bashh.org/ documents/118/118.pdf].

6 Ross J, Judlin P, Nilas L. European guideline for the management of pelvic inflammatory disease. *Int J STD AIDs* 2007;18:662–6.

7 British National Formulary [bnf.org/bnf/bnf/60/3944. htm?q=quinolones tendon damage&t=search&ss=text&p=1].

8 Royal College of Obstetricians and Gynaecologists. *Acute pelvic inflammatory disease (PID): tests and treatment. Information for you.* London: RCOG; 2010 [www.rcog.org.uk/ acute-pelvic-inflammatory-disease-tests-treatment].

9 National Chlamydia Screening Programme. What is the NCSP? What are the aims of the NCSP? 2010 [www.chlamydiascreening.nhs.uk/ps/what_is/aims.html].

10 Salisbury C, Macleod J, Egger M, McCarthy A, Patel R, Holloway A, et al. Opportunistic and systematic screening for chlamydia: a study of consultations by young adults in general practice. *Br J Gen Pract* 2006;56:99–103

11 Lavelle S J, Jones K E, Mallinson H, Webb A M. Finding, confirming, and managing gonorrhoea in a population screened for chlamydia using the Gen-Probe Aptima Combo2 assay. *Sex Transm Infect* 2006;82:221–4.

12 Hopwood J, Mallinson H. Chlamydia testing in community clinics – a focus for accurate sexual health care. *Br J Fam Plann* 1995;21:87–90

13 Gleave T, Hopwood J, Mallinson H. Management of Chlamydia trachomatis in a women's hospital: a review of current practice. *J Fam Plann Reprod Health Care* 2001:27: 161–2.

14 National Screening Committee. *First Report of the National Screening Committee. Health Departments of the United Kingdom.* London; National Screening Committee, Department of Health; 1998 [www.dh.gov.uk/prod_consum_ dh/groups/dh_digitalassets/documents/digitalasset/ dh_084456.pdf].

15 Sylvan S, Christenson B. Increase in Chlamydia trachomatis infection in Sweden: time for new strategies. *Arch Sex Behav* 2008;37:362–4.

16 Scottish Intercollegiate Guidelines Network. National Clinical Practice Guideline No. 109: *Management of genital Chlamydia trachomatis infection.* Edinburgh: SIGN; 2009 [www.sign.ac.uk/guidelines/fulltext/109/index.html].

17 Turner K M E, Adams E J, Lamontagne D S, Emmett L, Baster K, Edmunds W J. Modelling the effectiveness of chlamydia screening in England. *Sex Transm Infect* 2006;82:496–502.

18 Adams E J, Turner K M, Edmunds W J. The cost effectiveness of opportunistic chlamydia screening in England. *Sex Transm Infect* 2007;83:267–74.

19 Low N, Eggar M, Sterne J A, Harbord R M, Ibrahim F, Lindblom B, et al. Incidence of severe reproductive tract complications associated with diagnosed genital chlamydial infection: the Uppsala Women's Cohort Study. *Sex Transm Infect* 2006;82:212–18.

16

Diagnosis and management of haemorrhagic and septic shock

Caroline Cormack and Natasha Curran

Introduction

Shock is a systemic disorder affecting multiple organ systems. Its early recognition and prompt treatment are very important as there is a direct correlation between the duration and severity of tissue hypoperfusion and poor outcome. This chapter describes the pathophysiology of haemorrhagic and septic shock, early diagnosis and principles of effective management.

Definition and mechanism of shock

Shock is a state of compromised tissue perfusion that causes cellular hypoxia. It is defined as a syndrome initiated by acute hypoperfusion leading to tissue hypoxia and vital organ dysfunction. During shock, perfusion is insufficient to meet the metabolic demands of the tissues and anaerobic metabolism occurs. This is unsustainable and, if not corrected, will progress to cellular dysfunction, cell death and end organ damage. The progressive chain of events that occurs as shock develops is summarised in Figure 16.1.

Recognition of shock

Prompt stabilisation of the woman's condition and treatment of the underlying cause of the shock can avoid the rapidly spiralling deterioration that leads to cell damage and, ultimately, death. The recognition of shock is clinical and depends on identification of the cluster of subtle signs associated with the development of tissue hypoxia and dysfunction. Tachypnoea and tachycardia are often early signs of shock, followed by hypotension and poor urine output. Only once shock has progressed some way will the patient also show the classic picture of pale, clammy skin, cool peripheries and an altered level of consciousness. The altered physiology of a pregnant woman may obscure the early signs of developing shock, making its recognition and early treatment even more difficult.

FIGURE 16.1 **Flow diagram illustrating the progressive chain of events that occurs as shock develops**

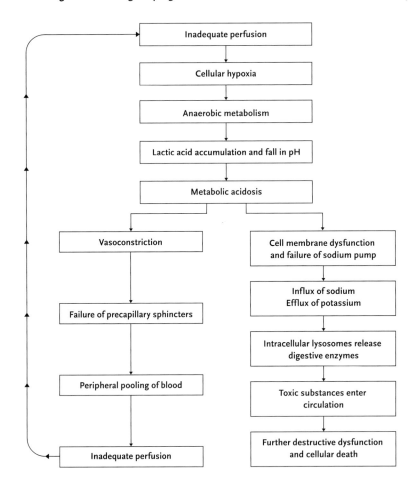

The reports of the Confidential Enquiries into Maternal Deaths in the United Kingdom have shown that failure to recognise that a woman was developing shock and late, inadequate or inappropriate therapeutic measures have contributed to the deaths of several women. One of the key recommendations in recent reports is that all NHS trusts should adopt a modified early warning system to help in the timely recognition, treatment and referral of women who have or who are developing critical conditions.[1]

Early warning systems are recommended in the monitoring of all acutely ill patients in hospital in the UK.[2] These systems are widely used in medical and surgical practice and are based on the monitoring of five simple variables: mental function, heart rate, systolic blood pressure, respiratory rate and temperature. Hourly urine output may be included if the woman is catheterised.

If the measured physiological variables exceed set parameters, medical attention or intervention is triggered. The parameters set in standard early warning systems are well established but do not take into account the changes that occur in the cardiovascular and respiratory systems during pregnancy. Therefore, if these parameters are used in a pregnant woman, they may trigger unnecessary action. Studies are currently being undertaken to establish what parameters should be adopted for use in early pregnancy and in labour[3] to trigger initial medical review and treatment and, if no improvement, referral to critical care or an outreach team. Until data are available as to the best parameters to use in early pregnancy, it seems sensible that standard early warning systems should be adopted and, if necessary, modified by the individual hospitals (Figure 16.2).

Management of shock

The management of shock is aimed at stabilising the woman while diagnosing and treating the underlying cause. In early pregnancy the causes of shock may be directly related to the pregnancy or may be coincidental, for example due to trauma or extragenital infection (Table 16.1).

Haemorrhagic shock

Haemorrhage may be classified by the volume of blood lost. The typical changes in vital signs associated with each volume of blood loss and typical transfusion requirements are shown in Table 16.2.

TABLE 16.1 **Causes of haemorrhage and sepsis in early pregnancy**

	Cause of haemorrhage	Source of sepsis
Directly related to pregnancy	Ectopic pregnancy	Infected retained products of conception
	Miscarriage	Septic miscarriage
	Ruptured corpus luteum cyst	Instrumentation of genitourinary tract
		Intravaginal mifepristone (*Clostridium sordellii* consistent with toxic shock)
Coincidental	Trauma	Urinary tract infection/pyelopephritis
	Postoperative bleeding	Intra-abdominal abscess
	Other source of bleeding (e.g. gastric ulcer)	Respiratory tract infection
		Central venous pressure line

FIGURE 16.2 **Example of an early warning system used at University College Hospital, London, Heart Hospital and the National Hospital for Neurology and Neurosurgery**

PARAMETERS FOR LOW LEVEL RESPONSE

Nurse-in-charge must be informed if:

RR / min	<10	>20
HR /min	<60	>90
SBP mmHg	<100	>160
Temp °C	<36	>38
Urine output	<30ml / hr for 2 consecutive hours (in a catheterised patient)	

Increasing oxygen requirements to keep oxygen saturations at prescribed target

Change in mental status / New or increasing drowsiness or confusion

 – at NHNN any change in mental status requires review by doctor (adverse clinical signs)
– any patients with head injury should follow NICE guidelines

Any concern about patient e.g. chest pain, colour change

The standard response for any patient exhibiting the above criteria will be to inform the nurse in charge, assess patient, and increase the frequency of observations.

Remember **ABCDE** approach.

Prompts for nurse-in-charge:

- ☑ Review previous observations
- ☑ What is normal for the patient?
- ☑ What is the trend?
- ☑ Review the fluid balance
- ☑ Do observations / fluid balance need to be more frequent?
- ☑ Should patient be on neuro obs? (if change in mental status)
- ☑ Do you need to:
  - Check the blood sugar?
  - 12 lead ECG?
  - Dipstick urine / MSU?
- ☑ Does a doctor need to review the patient?
- ☑ Have you documented your action?

If patient condition does not improve inform medical staff for review.

Is the patient meeting PERT call criteria (UCH / HH) or adverse clinical signs (NHNN)?

Consider sepsis if patient has 2 or more of the following:

RR >20
T >38 or <36 °C
HR >90
altered consciousness
hyperglycaemia (but not diabetic)
WCC >12 OR <4 × 10⁹/ L

Sepsis

ABCDE = airway, breathing, circulation, disability, exposure | ECG = electrocardiogram | HH = Heart Hospital | HR = heart rate | MSU = mid-stream urine | NHNN= National Hospital for Neurology and Neurosurgery | NICE = National Institute for Health and Clinical Excellence | PERT = patient emergency response team | SBP = systolic blood pressure | T = temperature | UCH = University College Hospital | WCC = white cell count. Reproduced with permission.

TABLE 16.2 **Classification of haemorrhage and typical resuscitation requirements**

Class	Volume (ml)	Blood volume (%)	Vital signs	Resuscitation requirements
I	750	<15	No change	Fluid resuscitation not typical
II	750–1500	15–30	Tachycardia Narrowed pulse Peripheral vasoconstriction Pallor	Volume resuscitation with crystalloid or colloid Blood transfusion not usually necessary
III	1500–2000	30–40	Tachycardia Low blood pressure Poor capillary refill Mental status worsens	Fluid resuscitation with crystalloid or colloid and blood transfusion usually necessary
IV	>2000	>40	Limit of body's compensation reached	Aggressive resuscitation required to prevent death

The aim is to resuscitate the woman while gathering information to allow the source of blood loss to be diagnosed so that it can be stopped, surgically if necessary. The resuscitation guidelines recommended in the UK are drawn up by the Resuscitation Council (UK).[4] They use an ABC (airway, breathing and circulation) format and should be familiar to all hospital doctors.

It is important to call early for help from other teams, such as anaesthetists, the intensive therapy unit and accident and emergency, because there is much to be done and the woman will remain at risk from the sequelae of massive transfusion even once the bleeding has stopped. If necessary, put out a 'fast bleep' or 'cardiac arrest' call.

Oxygen

Give the woman oxygen. With fewer red blood cells available to carry oxygen to the tissues, supplemental oxygen will help to reduce tissue hypoxia.

Fluid resuscitation

Circulatory resuscitation requirements depend on the volume of blood lost, as shown in Table 16.2. Blood loss of up to approximately 2 litres can usually be managed with infusion of warm clear fluids (colloid or crystalloid) and packed red cells. Blood loss of greater than 2 litres requires urgent and aggressive management.

In early pregnancy a woman's circulation is hyperdynamic with reduced systemic vascular resistance. By 10 weeks of gestation, maternal cardiac output has increased by 30–50% as a result of increased heart rate and stroke volume. Some haemodilution will have occurred, although this does not reach its maximum until about 32 weeks of gestation. This means that physiological compensation for haemorrhage is reduced and transfusion may be required sooner.

It must be remembered that while most pregnant women are otherwise fit, coexisting medical conditions may make individual women less able to tolerate significant blood loss or aggressive fluid resuscitation. These women are very difficult to manage, especially if bleeding is sudden and unexpected.

If women have a massive haemorrhage, intravenous access must be secured with at least two wide-bore cannulae and fluid given. It is best if this fluid is warmed as enzyme systems such as the coagulation cascade work most efficiently at 37°C. However, resuscitation should not be delayed if warmed fluid is not immediately available.

Blood transfusion

Telephone the haematology department and initiate a 'massive haemorrhage alert'. Most hospitals will have a set of guidelines drawn up for this situation but, if you are unsure, cross-match six units of packed red cells urgently and send blood samples for a full blood count, coagulation screen and urea and electrolytes. It is rarely necessary to give a woman uncross-matched O negative blood.

Definitive haemostasis

Continually reassess the nature and volume of the blood loss, bearing in mind that it may be occult. Take steps to stop the bleeding, transferring the woman to theatre urgently if necessary.

Blood product administration

It is common for coagulation abnormalities to develop as a result of massive haemorrhage and transfusion. In severe cases the woman may develop disseminated intravascular coagulopathy. Coagulation abnormalities are treated with transfusion of blood products (fresh frozen plasma, cryoprecipitate and platelets) under the guidance of the on-call haematologist.

Recombinant factor VIIa is licensed for use only in congenital and acquired haemophilia, factor VII deficiency and Glanzmann's thromboasthenia. It has been used off-licence in the treatment of people with continuing severe haemorrhage despite attempts to correct coagulopathy and optimal attempts at management of haemostasis. In massive haemorrhage, recombinant factor VIIa is most effective if used early. There is some evidence that it may reduce the amount of blood products needed and the duration of subsequent mechanical ventilation and other critical care support. Advice from haematologists is needed before it is used.[5]

Septic shock

Sepsis is defined as documented or suspected infection associated with one or more of the symptoms and signs outlined in Table 16.3. Severe sepsis is sepsis associated with organ dysfunction, hypoperfusion or hypotension, such as septic shock (Table 16.4).

Women with sepsis are critically ill and require urgent and aggressive resuscitation. The response to treatment in this population is highly unpredictable and the mortality rate is high. Treatment is more likely to be effective, and severe sepsis avoided, if appropriate therapy is started early.

The goals of management are to resuscitate the woman and eliminate the underlying infection using appropriate antibiotics. A variety of supportive interventions in critical care may be required, for example mechanical ventilation and kidney dialysis, so it is advisable to involve other teams early.

The Surviving Sepsis Campaign[6] has drawn up guidelines for the management of sepsis and septic shock based on a review of the current literature by an international panel of experts. These guidelines recommend the use of clinical protocols for early resuscitation with the aim of achieving the following goals within the first 6 hours after diagnosis of sepsis:

- central venous pressure of 8–12 mmHg

- mean arterial pressure over 65 mmHg

- urine output over 0.5 ml/kg/hour

- central venous oxygen saturation over 70% or mixed venous oxygen saturation over 65%.

The following guidelines are for treatments that can be started immediately while the woman is on a general ward awaiting the arrival of critical care specialists. It must be remembered that there is a direct correlation between the duration and severity of tissue hypoperfusion and poor outcome, so there should be no delay in starting resuscitation.

Fluid therapy

If the woman is hypotensive, fluid resuscitation should begin immediately. Initially, give warmed fluid challenges of 1000 ml of crystalloids or 300–

TABLE 16.3 **Definition of sepsis based on clinical symptoms and signs**

Variables

General	Inflammatory	Other
Fever or hypothermia (core temperature <36°C or >38.3°C)	White cell count <4000 or >12 000/μl (or normal with >10% immature forms)	Mixed venous oxygen saturation >70% Cardiac index >3.5 litres/minute
Heart rate >90 beats/minute	C-reactive protein >2 standard deviations above normal value	
Tachypnoea	Procalcitonin >2 standard deviations above normal value	
Altered mental status		
Significant oedema or large positive fluid balance		
Hyperglycaemia (plasma glucose >6.7 mmol/l)		

500 ml of colloids over 30 minutes and check for haemodynamic improvement. Larger volumes may be required for the treatment of septic shock, but beware of overloading the woman with fluid.

It may be useful to insert a central venous line, but this must not delay resuscitation of the woman. Central venous pressure (CVP) monitoring will guide effective fluid therapy and warn of impending fluid overload as shown by rising cardiac filling pressures without haemodynamic improvement. The central venous pressure line can also be used to obtain central venous samples to monitor oxygenation. Other methods of monitoring cardiac output, for example oesophageal Doppler monitoring, may be used to guide and optimise fluid resuscitation in the critical care setting. In these cases, central venous pressure insertion during the initial resuscitation is less important if the woman is likely to be admitted to critical care soon.

Diagnosis

It is important to obtain appropriate cultures before starting antibiotics, provided this does not cause significant delay in giving them. At least two sets of blood cultures are advised, of which one should be taken through a fresh venous puncture. If any vascular access devices have been in place for more than 48 hours, a blood culture sample should be taken from each device. Other sites should be cultured as clinically indicated.

TABLE 16.4 **Signs of severe sepsis**

Variables

Organ dysfunction	Tissue perfusion	Haemodynamic
Arterial hypoxaemia	Hyperlactataemia (serum lactate >2 mmol/l)	Hypotension (mean systolic blood pressure <90 mmHg, mean arterial blood pressure <70 mmHg)
Acute oliguria (urine output <0.5 ml/kg/hour)		
Raised serum creatinine		
Coagulation abnormalities (INR > 1.5 or APTT > 60 seconds)		
Thrombocytopenia (platelet count <100/dl)		
Hyperbilirubinaemia (>35 mmol/l)		

APTT = activated partial thromboplastin time | INR = international normalised ratio.

Antimicrobial therapy

Begin intravenous antibiotics as early as possible, always within the first hour of recognising severe sepsis. Antibacterial agents should be used that cover the likely bacterial and fungal pathogens and that have good penetration to the presumed source of infection, in line with local guidelines, as likely pathogens and resistances can vary locally. The choice of antibiotics may be refined once a microbiological diagnosis has been made, and this choice should be reviewed daily to optimise efficacy, prevent resistance, avoid toxicity and minimise costs.

Blood product administration

It is common for women with severe sepsis to develop a coagulopathy and thrombocytopenia. If the woman is not actively bleeding and no invasive procedures are planned, she may be able to tolerate the abnormal laboratory clotting results. However, if the platelet count falls to 5×10^9 per litre, platelets should be given regardless of bleeding. If there is a significant risk of bleeding or if surgery or invasive procedures are planned, platelets will be needed to keep the count above 50×10^9 per litre. In these circumstances other teams such as critical care and haematology should be involved. Give red blood cells when haemoglobin is less than 7.0 g/dl, with the aim of achieving a target haemoglobin of 7.0–9.0 g/dl.[6]

Vasopressors

One of the stated goals of resuscitation is to achieve and maintain mean arterial pressure greater than or equal to 65 mmHg within the first 6 hours following the diagnosis of severe sepsis.[6] Mean arterial pressure is estimated as (systolic blood pressure + [2 × diastolic blood pressure]) ÷ 3. Cardiac function may be compromised as a result of the septic shock and women can easily become fluid-overloaded if they are given excessive volumes of fluid during resuscitation. In these circumstances an infusion of noradrenaline (norepinephrine) or dopamine via a central line is needed to achieve and maintain the desired mean arterial pressure; excessive fluid should be avoided. Women with these symptoms are clearly very unwell and require urgent admission to a critical care unit to start infusion of a vasopressor. Noradrenaline and dopamine are the vasopressors of choice in the treatment of septic shock. Noradrenaline may be combined with dobutamine when cardiac output is being measured. Adrenaline (epinephrine), phenylephrine and vasopressin are not recommended as first-line agents in the treatment of septic shock. Vasopressin may be considered for salvage therapy. Low-dose dopamine is not recommended for the purpose of renal protection. Dobutamine is recommended as the agent of choice to increase cardiac output, but should not be used for the purpose of increasing cardiac output above physiological levels.[6]

Other treatments

The following are other treatments that may be provided in the critical care setting during the management of a woman with septic shock. They are included here for completeness, but obstetric and gynaecology teams would not be expected to start these treatments as part of the initial resuscitation of a woman.

CORTICOSTEROIDS

Intravenous hydrocortisone can be used in women with septic shock if their hypotension remains poorly responsive to adequate fluid resuscitation and vasopressors. However, it should not be used to treat sepsis in the absence of shock unless the woman's endocrine or corticosteroid history warrants it.

GLUCOSE CONTROL

Intravenous insulin infusions can be used to control hyperglycaemia in women with severe sepsis. An infusion regimen that aims to keep the blood glucose below 10 mmol/l is recommended.[7] If tighter glycaemic control is the aim, for example 4–6 mmol/l, there is a greater risk of severe hypoglycaemia and the overall mortality rate in the intensive care unit is higher.

OTHER CONDITIONS

Women in critical care are at risk of developing stress ulcers and deep vein thrombosis. Prophylactic treatment for these conditions is usually given. It may be necessary for the woman to receive treatments such as mechanical ventilation and renal replacement therapy to support organ systems that have failed as a result of the septic shock while recovery has a chance to occur. Decisions regarding starting and stopping these treatments and others are usually taken by critical care specialists.

Conclusion

Haemorrhagic and septic shock are difficult to diagnose and manage in early pregnancy. Early warning scoring systems can help in making the initial diagnosis, allowing treatment to be commenced early and a crisis to be averted. If shock develops it will affect multiple organ systems, so advice from critical care and other teams should be sought early. Nonetheless, it is vital for staff on the general ward to act quickly to provide adequate and appropriate resuscitation and definitive treatment of the underlying problem as soon as possible. This will minimise the duration and severity of tissue hypoperfusion and improve the chance of a good outcome.

References

1 Clutton-Brook T. Critical Care. In: *Saving Mothers' Lives: Reviewing maternal deaths to make motherhood safer 2003–2005. The Seventh Report of the Confidential Enquiries into Maternal Deaths in the United Kingdom*. London: Confidential Enquiry into Maternal and Child Health; 2007 [www.cmace. org.uk/getattachment/927cf18a-735a-47a0-9200-cdea103781c7/ Saving-Mothers--Lives-2003-2005_full.aspx].

2 Centre for Clinical Practice, National Institute for Health and Clinical Excellence. *NICE clinical guideline 50. Quick reference guide. Acutely ill patients in hospital. Recognition of and response to acute illness in adults in hospital*. London: NICE; 2007 [www.nice.org.uk/nicemedia/pdf/ CG50QuickRefGuide.pdf].

3 Swanton R D, Al-Rawi S, Wee M Y. A national survey of obstetric early warning systems in the United Kingdom. *Int J Obstet Anesth* 2009;18:253–7.

4 Resuscitation Council (UK). *Advanced Life Support*. 5th ed. London: Resuscitation Council (UK); 2008.

5 Levi M, Peters M, Büller H R. Efficacy and safety of recombinant factor VIIa for treatment of severe bleeding: a systematic review. *Crit Care Med* 2005;33:883–90.

6 Dellinger R P, Levy M M, Carlet J M, Bion J, Parker M M, Jaeschke R, et al. Surviving Sepsis Campaign: international guidelines for management of severe sepsis and septic shock: 2008. *Crit Care Med* 2008;36:296–327. Erratum in: *Crit Care Med* 2008;36:1394–6.

7 NICE-SUGAR Study Investigators, Finfer S, Chittock D R, Su S Y, Blair D, Foster D, Dhingra V, et al. Intensive versus conventional glucose control in critically ill patients. *N Engl J Med* 2009;360:1283–97.

17 Role of minimally invasive surgery in acute gynaecology

Christy Burden and Sanjay Vyas

Introduction

Minimally invasive surgery is increasingly being used to diagnose and treat women presenting with acute gynaecological disorders. Laparotomy was previously the standard treatment for acute gynaecological emergencies such as ruptured ectopic pregnancy or ovarian cyst accidents. In most women the diagnosis was first confirmed by laparoscopy before open surgery was carried out. As the technology and surgical experience have improved, more women have been managed exclusively using laparoscopic surgery. New instruments have been developed that allow safe manipulation of the pelvic organs. Procedures such as irrigation, haemostasis and intra-abdominal suturing can be carried out without the need for open surgery. Minimally invasive surgery can now be used for both the diagnosis and treatment of many acute gynaecological conditions.[1] Laparoscopic surgery can therefore be limited to a diagnostic procedure if the diagnosis is in doubt or expanded into an operative procedure once the diagnosis has been made and immediate treatment is required.

Benefits and risks of minimally invasive surgery

Laparoscopic surgery is associated with reduced postoperative pain, intra-operative blood loss, wound complications, adhesions, length of hospital stay and recovery time compared with laparotomy.[2] Additional benefits include better visualisation and more precision while operating. Laparoscopic management of ectopic pregnancies has been proved to be advantageous in terms of treatment outcomes, postoperative adhesions, hospital stay, cost and effects on long-term fertility.[3–5] Laparoscopic surgery can also be used to treat ectopic pregnancy in obese women.[6] Laparoscopy is highly accurate in the diagnosis of ectopic pregnancy and its use should be encouraged in the emergency setting when the diagnosis is uncertain.[7]

Increasingly, other gynaecological emergencies can now also be managed laparoscopically. It has been shown that laparoscopic surgery is superior to

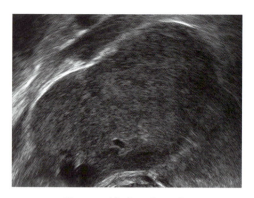

FIGURE 17.1 Ultrasound finding of a swollen oedematous ovary in a young woman complaining of acute abdominal pain is highly suggestive of torsion

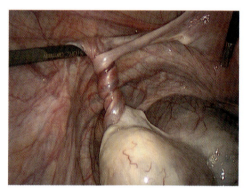

FIGURE 17.2 Laparoscopic finding of ovarian torsion in a woman with a history of acute lower abdominal pain

Courtesy of Mr George Pandis, University College Hospital, London.

laparotomy in the treatment of ovarian torsion, even in pregnant women.[8,9] Laparoscopy can also be useful to confirm the diagnosis of pelvic inflammatory disease (PID) and to exclude other pelvic pathology.[10] Other benefits include the ability to take microbiological samples to facilitate appropriate antibiotic therapy and drainage of a pelvic abscess.

The disadvantages of laparoscopic surgery include increased complication rates, particularly ureteric damage, and a longer operating time. The use of laparoscopy in haemodynamically unstable women with a haemoperitoneum is controversial but not contraindicated.[11-13]

Preoperative assessment

History

Adequate preoperative assessment is essential prior to any laparoscopic treatment of a gynaecological emergency. Important factors in the woman's history include her age, the date of her last menstrual period, pain, bleeding, the presence of comorbidities and a history of previous surgery and pelvic infection. The differential diagnosis includes ectopic pregnancy, ovarian or adnexal accidents (torsion, haemorrhage and rupture) and PID with or without pelvic abscess. Degenerating leiomyomas are also rare causes of acute pain. Endometriosis and pelvic adhesions usually cause chronic pain, but may present acutely. Pelvic ultrasonography is an essential preoperative investigation. Computed tomography and magnetic resonance imaging are rarely of benefit except in the exclusion of other pathologies.

Presenting symptoms

Pelvic pain
Pelvic pain is typically caused by ovarian cyst accidents, which include rupture, haemorrhage and torsion. Ovarian torsion is defined as partial or complete rotation of the ovarian vascular pedicle causing obstruction initially to the venous outflow and later to the arterial inflow as well (Figures 17.1 and 17.2).

Torsion of a normal ovary and adnexa may sometimes occur.[12] Benign dermoid cysts are a common cause of torsion. Malignant tumours rarely present with torsion as they are usually fixed by adhesions to the surrounding pelvic structures. Clinical features associated with torsion are variable, but often include anorexia, nausea and vomiting as well as abdominal pain. On examination, women with adnexal torsion may be systemically unwell with peripheral vasoconstriction, tachypnoea and decreased oxygen saturation with metabolic acidosis. Suspected torsion should always be managed surgically.

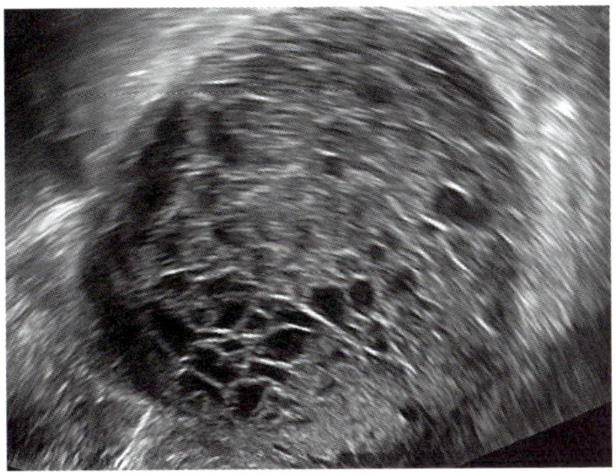

Ovarian cyst rupture and haemorrhage usually occur in association with physiological (functional) cysts. Most are self-limiting (Figure 17.3). Laparoscopy may be required if the diagnosis is uncertain and/or there is a lack of resolution of symptoms or signs of haemodynamic instability (Figure 17.4). Clinical features include pain, raised pulse rate, normal temperature and normal blood pressure with focal tenderness on abdominal palpation. Dermoid and endometriotic cysts may also rupture. These cases are rare, but may be associated with severe peritonitis and systemic illness.[12]

Haemorrhagic shock

Ectopic pregnancy remains one of the most common causes of intraperitoneal bleeding and haemorrhagic shock. However, the majority of women with ectopic pregnancies present with gradual intra-abdominal bleeding and may remain haemodynamically stable despite developing a large haemoperitoneum of 1000–1500 ml.[11] Women who have secondary bleeding postoperatively or massive bleeding from a ruptured ovarian cyst will present with similar symptoms.

Infection

PID usually occurs because of an ascending infection affecting the uterus, the fallopian tubes and the surrounding pelvic structures. However, the clinical presentation varies and the diagnosis is often delayed. If PID is inadequately treated, a tubo-ovarian pelvic abscess may develop. Women with a tubo-ovarian abscess typically present with abdominal pain, irregular vaginal bleeding and

FIGURE 17.3 **A case of haemorrhagic ovarian cyst**

The ovary is enlarged with a cyst that contains fresh blood clots.

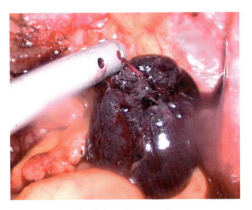

FIGURE 17.4 **A blood clot adjacent to the ovary in a woman with acute pain owing to a ruptured functional cyst**

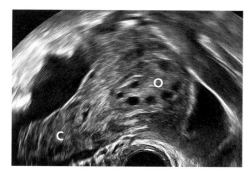

FIGURE 17.5 **Ultrasound findings in a woman with a large haematoperitoneum**

The ovary (O) is surrounded by a large blood clot (C).

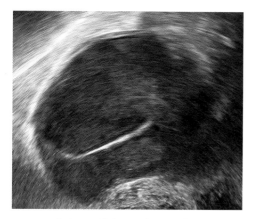

FIGURE 17.6 **A case of a large subacute tubo-ovarian abscess containing typical low-echogenicity fluid**

dyspareunia with or without fever. The abdomen is tender on palpation with rebound and guarding. Vaginal examination often reveals a mucopurulent discharge, while bimanual examination may give rise to suspicion of an adnexal mass.

Clinical examination and diagnostic tests

The clinical examination involves assessing signs of haemodynamic instability (blood pressure, pulse and urine output), sepsis (temperature, oxygen saturation, peripheral vasoconstriction and acidosis) and presence of abdominal peritonism (abdominal distension, rebound tenderness, guarding and bowel sounds). A vaginal examination should be undertaken to check for cervical excitation, adnexal tenderness or presence of a mass.

A urinary pregnancy test should always be performed in women of reproductive age with abdominal pain. A full blood count, urea and electrolytes, C-reactive protein, liver function tests, beta-human chorionic gonadotrophin hormone and coagulation screens should be taken. Serum CA125 should not usually be taken as it is particularly non-specific in the acute setting and in women of reproductive age. CA125 can be raised with any cause of peritonitis, including haemorrhage, cyst rupture and infection, as well as menstruation, fibroids and endometriosis. The white blood cell count may be raised in torsion but may also occur because of infection, pelvic abscess and appendicitis. Urinary dipstick, microscopy and culture should be undertaken to assess for blood, nitrites and leucocytes to rule out urinary infection or calculus. Arterial blood gases may reveal hypoxia and acidosis in acutely unwell women. If PID is suspected, endocervical and vaginal swabs should be taken.

Pelvic ultrasonography should be a first-line investigation in acutely ill women. In cases of ovarian torsion, an ultrasound scan may show an enlarged oedematous ovary with peripheral displacement of follicles. Colour Doppler may demonstrate a lack of arterial or venous flow and a twisted vascular pedicle. Nevertheless, these findings are variable and are not always diagnostic.[12] The typical appearance of a haemorrhagic cyst on ultrasound scan is an enlarged ovary containing mixed echoes in a reticular pattern. The appearance of a ruptured ovarian cyst on ultrasound is less typical and often only the presence of free fluid in the pouch of Douglas is an indication that a cyst rupture may have occurred (Figure 17.5). Women of reproductive age commonly have small physiological cysts and caution needs to be taken in attributing the symptoms of an acutely unwell woman to these findings on ultrasound. Ultrasound diagnosis of ectopic pregnancy is discussed in Chapter 9.

A tubo-ovarian abscess can be seen as a complex cystic adnexal mass with thick irregular walls, septations and internal echoes on ultrasound scan (Figure 17.6). Computed tomography and magnetic resonance imaging can aid in diagnosis, but the evidence for these two imaging methods is limited.[9]

Preparation for surgery

It is vital that women receive appropriate resuscitation before surgery commences.[13] The airway should be assessed as patent and oxygen should be administered. It is important to liaise with the anaesthetist or an intensive care doctor and involve them in the care of the woman at an early stage, especially if the woman's airway may be compromised. The woman's breathing should be assessed. A respiratory rate above 20 breaths per minute can be indicative of a respiratory problem or worsening metabolic acidosis. The woman's cardiovascular status should also be examined. Heart rate and capillary refill should be assessed and blood pressure taken. A tachycardic woman who is hypotensive is potentially in hypovolaemic shock.

Intravenous access should be obtained and bloods sent at the same time. If large blood loss is anticipated, two large-bore (16-gauge or above) cannulae should be placed and a cross-match taken on top of other routine bloods. An electrocardiogram, chest X-ray and arterial blood gases may be undertaken depending on the clinical situation. The woman needs to be kept warm and her temperature should be taken. The woman may need to receive fluid replacement if there is evidence of hypovolaemia. If the woman is septic, broad-spectrum intravenous antibiotics should be commenced with the involvement of microbiologists. The woman's Glasgow Coma Scale score, which is dependent upon verbal, motor and eye responses, can also be assessed. A score of less than 8 means there is a risk of airway problems and the airway may need to be secured. Urinary catheterisation should be performed to allow accurate assessment of the fluid balance. Further invasive monitoring such as a central or arterial line may be required.

BOX 17.1 **Essential equipment for operative laparoscopic surgery**

- 10 mm 0° laparoscope
- Umbilical port and three access ports
- Suction/irrigation
- Maryland grasper (with monopolar diathermy attached)
- Manhes grasper (toothed grasper)
- Atraumatic grasper
- Laparoscopic scissors
- Bipolar forceps
- Tripolar forceps
- Endoloop
- Laparoscopic needle holder and sutures

Planning the operation

The team required for any laparoscopic procedure must be defined. This should include the surgeon, anaesthetist, surgical assistant, anaesthesia assistant, scrub nurse, operating department practitioner and runner. The same people would be involved in a laparotomy, should the laparoscopy need to be converted to open surgery. Good communication is essential to ensure that the urgency of the operation is determined and the appropriate operating theatre is chosen to undertake the procedure. The essential equipment for laparoscopic procedures is listed in Box 17.1.

Surgical techniques

The woman should be placed in the Lloyd–Davies position, with her buttocks well down the operating table. A Foley catheter should be placed in the bladder and a uterine manipulator in the uterus, unless there is the possibility of an intrauterine pregnancy. The surgeon should supervise the positioning of the woman to ensure that her uterus can be manipulated with ease, as poor positioning at this stage will require repositioning later, leading to delays in providing effective treatment.

In women with evidence of significant intra-abdominal haemorrhage, blood should first be removed using suction irrigation. This will also facilitate identification of the source of the bleeding (Figures 17.7 and 17.8). Once the bleeding point has been identified, the bleeding can be arrested using various techniques, including bipolar/tripolar coagulation, clip application, endoloop or suturing. Ectopic pregnancies can be managed by salpingotomy or salpingectomy depending on the gestational age, the severity of the tubal damage and the woman's desire for future fertility.

Surgery for pelvic infection and abscess historically included transabdominal drainage and unilateral or bilateral oophorectomy. Although these procedures had high cure rates, they had adverse effects on future fertility and ovarian reserve. The aim of surgery involves lysis of adhesions, drainage of the abscess, excision of infected and necrotic tissue and irrigation of the peritoneal cavity. It has been shown that operative laparoscopy involving drainage of adnexal abscesses is a safe and effective procedure.[10,14] One study compared intraoperative and postoperative complications in women who had laparoscopic incision of the abscess cavity and lavage only with women who had laparoscopic salpingectomy or salpingoophorectomy.[15] There were significantly lower complication rates with the organ-saving procedures.

Ovarian torsion was previously managed with ovarian cystectomy or oophorectomy when the ovary looked engorged or ischaemic. However, laparoscopic detorsion with or without cystectomy or ovariopexy is now commonly used, and has been shown to preserve ovarian function in 91–100% of cases.[12] The macroscopic appearance of the ovary, unless gangrene is present, is unreliable in predicting ovarian tissue viability. Adnexal necrosis needing repeat intervention for peritonitis has been seen following detorsion, but is rare. Follicular development on ultrasound scan can be used to assess ovarian viability following detorsion. Postmenopausal women with torsion should normally be managed with bilateral oophorectomy.

The findings of adhesions or endometriosis at laparoscopy are common. In our experience these conditions rarely cause acute abdominal pain. Therefore, our recommendation in an emergency operation would be to leave them alone and not perform adhesiolysis, excision or ablation, provided that the rest of the pelvis has been adequately examined at laparoscopy. If on inspection the pelvic organs appear normal, a careful examination of the rest of the abdominal cavity should be performed. Further management depends on the findings of the examination. A general surgical consultation may be needed.

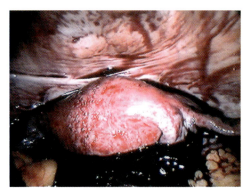

FIGURE 17.7 **Large haematoperitoneum found at laparoscopy in a case of suspected ectopic pregnancy**

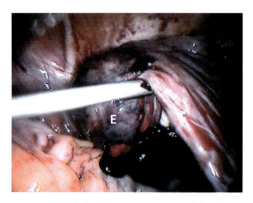

FIGURE 17.8 **A left tubal ectopic pregnancy (E) is clearly visible after aspiration of the haemoperitoneum**

Performing laparoscopic surgery on an acutely ill woman may have implications for respiratory and cardiovascular function. The creation of a pneumoperitoneum will exert pressure against the diaphragm and abdominal vasculature, which may reduce cardiac output. This can be reversed by placing the woman in the Trendelenburg position. It should be borne in mind that this position can cause difficulties with ventilation, so it may be safer to adopt a limited Trendelenburg position; however, this may limit visualisation of the pelvis owing to the presence of the small bowel. In these cases, the bowel would need to be carefully lifted out of the pelvis using instruments introduced into the abdomen through the accessory ports. A pneumoperitoneum may also trigger a parasympathetic vasovagal reflex resulting in lowering of the pulse rate despite hypotension. However, an increase in intra-abdominal pressure will to some extent tamponade the small blood vessels, helping to slow down blood loss.

After insertion of the primary port, the laparoscope should be introduced cautiously so that it does not come into contact with the blood in the peritoneal cavity. This will ensure a good view and avoid delays in securing haemostasis. If the pelvic organs are obscured by blood, the blood can be removed by suction irrigation and the bleeding point identified. Alternatively, the uterus can be acutely anteflexed by the uterine manipulator to identify the bleeding point on the fallopian tube in cases of ruptured ectopic pregnancies.

An important consideration is the surgeon's skill at laparoscopic surgery. It is essential that the surgeon is able to ensure haemostasis in a short time. To this end, it is crucial that the surgeon is aware of his or her level of competence and limitations. Open surgery must be considered if the surgeon does not consider that he or she possesses the necessary skills to perform the laparoscopic procedure quickly, safely and effectively. It is also essential that the surgical team and theatre staff are familiar with operative requirements and instruments so that slow set-up and lack of equipment do not delay an emergency surgical procedure. The surgical team and theatre staff must also be able to swiftly troubleshoot any equipment failures to avoid further prolonging the operating time. Performing a greater number of elective laparoscopic procedures will not only increase the surgeon's skill but will also provide the rest of the surgical team with greater familiarity with the equipment and procedures, improving performance in an emergency setting.

Postoperative care

Postoperative care should involve close observation of vital signs and the use of a catheter to assess fluid balance. This is especially important if the woman is septic or is hypovolaemic from excessive blood loss. A drain may be inserted to ascertain any continuing bleeding or to drain pus. A blood transfusion may be required if the woman is severely anaemic or haemodynamically unstable. All women should be encouraged to mobilise early if appropriate and be considered for thromboprophylaxis with compression stockings and low-molecular-weight heparin. Women may require postoperative care in the intensive care or high-dependency unit depending on their clinical condition.

Conclusions

In experienced hands, laparoscopic surgery is an effective and safe method for the treatment of acute gynaecological conditions. A thorough preoperative assessment is required with adequate resuscitation. Emergency laparoscopy can be performed in women who are obese or in the presence of a significant haemoperitoneum. However, the critical factor in determining the most appropriate surgical approach is the skill of the operating surgeon, anaesthetist and theatre team. Familiarity with procedures and equipment is essential to ensure prompt and successful treatment of gynaecological emergencies using laparoscopic surgery. There are many benefits of laparoscopic over open surgery, and the increased use of emergency laparoscopic surgery is advantageous not only to individual women but to their families and to wider society as well.

References

1 Magos AL, Baumann R, Turnbull AC. Managing gynaecological emergencies with laparoscopy. *BMJ* 1989;299:371–4.

2 Warren O, Kinross J, Paraskeva P, Darzi A. Emergency laparoscopy – current best practice. *World J Emerg Surg* 2006;1:24.

3 Murphy A A, Nager C W, Wujek J J, Kettel L M, Torp V A, Chin H G. Operative laparoscopy versus laparotomy for the management of ectopic pregnancy: a prospective trial. *Fertil Steril* 1992;57:1180–5.

4 Lundorff P,Thorburn J, Lindblom B. Fertility outcome after conservative surgical treatment of ectopic pregnancy evaluated in a randomized trial. *Fertil Steril* 1992;57: 998–1002.

5 Gray D, Thorburn J, Lundorff P, Strandell A, Lindblom B. A cost-effectiveness study of a randomised trial of laparoscopy versus laparotomy for ectopic pregnancy. *Lancet* 1995;345:1139–43.

6 Hsu S, Mitwally M F, Aly A, Al-Saheh M, Batt R E, Yeh J. Laparoscopic management of tubal ectopic pregnancy in obese women. *Fertil Steril* 2004;81:198–202.

7 Golash V, Wilson P D. Early laparoscopy as a routine procedure in the management of acute abdominal pain: a review of 1,320 patients. *Surg Endosc* 2005;19:882–5.

8 Yuen P M, Yu K M, Yip S K, Lau W C, Rogers M S, Chang A. A randomized prospective study of laparoscopy and laparotomy in the management of benign ovarian masses. *Am J Obstet Gynecol* 1997;177:109–14.

9 Mais V, Ajossa S, Piras B, Marongiu D, Guerriero S, Melis G B. Treatment of nonendometriotic benign adnexal cysts: a randomized comparison of laparoscopy and laparotomy. *Obstet Gynecol* 1995;86:770–4.

10 Granberg S, Gjelland K, Elkerhovd E. The management of pelvic abscess. *Best Pract Res Clin Obstet Gynaecol* 2009;23:667–8.

11 Agdi M, Tulandi T. Surgical treatment of ectopic pregnancy. *Best Pract Res Clin Obstet Gynaecol* 2009; 519–27.

12 Bottomly C, Bourne T. Diagnosis and management of ovarian cyst accidents. *Best Pract Res Clin Obstet Gynaecol* 2009;23:711–24.

13 Centre for Clinical Practice, National Institute for Health and Clinical Excellence (NICE). *NICE clinical guideline 50: Acutely ill patients in hospital. Recognition of and response to acute illness in adults in hospital*. London: NICE; 2007 [guidance.nice.org.uk/CG50].

14 Raiga J, Canis M, Le Bouedec G, Glowaczower E, Pouly J L, Mage G, et al. Laparoscopic management of adnexal abscesses: consequences for fertility. *Fertil Steril* 1996;66:712–7.

15 Buchweitz O, Malik E, Kressin P, Meyhoefer-Malik A, Diedrich K. Laparoscopic management of tubo-ovarian abscess: retrospective analysis of 60 cases. *Surg Endosc* 2000;14:948–50.

Index